Some of the most commonly asked questions about hypertension:

• Do I still need to worry about strokes if neither of my parents is hypertensive or suffered a stroke?

• I have frequent headaches that are sometimes so painful that I get dizzy and feel nauseated. Am I suffering from hypertension?

• I had a stroke about three months ago. I'm recovering at home and wonder if it's possible for me to resume sexual relations with my partner?

• Will having a glass of wine or a cocktail every evening after work relax me enough to lower my blood pressure?

• My father and my paternal uncle both suffered strokes. What are my chances of having a stroke?

You'll find the answers to these and many other questions in this lifesaving book.

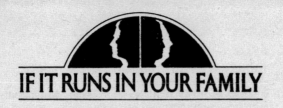

IF IT RUNS IN YOUR FAMILY

HYPERTENSION

REDUCING YOUR RISK

James M. Salander, M.D., F.A.C.S.,
and Suzanne LeVert

Foreword by Randall M. Zusman, M.D.,
Massachusetts General Hospital

Developed by The Philip Lief Group, Inc.

BANTAM BOOKS
NEW YORK · TORONTO · LONDON · SYDNEY · AUCKLAND

This book is not intended as a substitute for the medical advice of physicians. The reader should regularly consult a physician in matters relating to his or her health and particularly with respect to any symptoms that may require diagnosis or medical attention. Readers should also speak with their own doctors about their own individual needs before starting any diet or fitness program. Consulting one's personal physician about diet and exercise is especially important if the reader is on any medication or is already under medical care for any illness.

IF IT RUNS IN YOUR FAMILY: HYPERTENSION

A Bantam Book / November 1993

ISBN 0–553–56381–5

Published simultaneously in the United States and Canada

Bantam Books are published by Bantam Books, a division of Bantam Doubleday Dell Publishing Group, Inc. Its trademark, consisting of the words "Bantam Books" and the portrayal of a rooster, is Registered in U.S. Patent and Trademark Office and in other countries. Marca Registrada. Bantam Books, 1540 Broadway, New York, New York 10036.

PRINTED IN THE UNITED STATES OF AMERICA

OPM   0 9 8 7 6 5 4 3 2 1

Dedicated to my family with love and appreciation for teaching me respect for people of all ages and how to help them with their problems.

—J.M.S

Contents

Foreword

During the last two decades, the number of Americans dying from myocardial infarctions (heart attacks) and cerebrovascular accidents (strokes) has decreased significantly. Unfortunately, the number of people experiencing these medical emergencies has not decreased as much as we would like. We have, however, been able to prevent acute deaths in patients experiencing these events through the development of the following:

- Coronary care units and neurological intensive care units.
- Medications to treat what might otherwise be a fatal cardiac arrhythmia.
- Sophisticated cardiac pacemakers that sustain the heartbeat in those with inadequate heart rates.
- Medications that open blood vessels, thereby limiting danger to patients whose hearts might other-

wise be strained to the point that they could not sustain life.

- Medications that prevent the death of brain tissue, the loss of which would lead to severe neurologic impairment.

Learning to manage these medical catastrophies is an important part of improving the health of the American public, but an equally, perhaps more important aspect of health care is the control and prevention of those risk factors that lead to vascular disease. Diseases of the heart and blood vessels numerically exceed any other cause of death in Americans, despite the many advances in health care. The risk factors for the development of cardiovascular disease have been established through long-term epidemiologic follow-up studies such as that initiated in Framingham, a small community in Massachusetts.

Among the risk factors that have been identified is high blood pressure, or hypertension. The use of anti-hypertensive therapy over the last twenty years has significantly reduced the incidence of stroke but has not significantly reduced the incidence of heart attack. These findings have led cardiologists to consider a multiple risk factor approach to the assessment of the cardiovascular risk of their patients. We now recognize that among the risk factors for the development of vascular disease are those that are not modifiable, for example, aging, being male, and having a family history of premature vascular disease and atherosclerosis. However, modifiable risk factors include control of blood pressure and cholesterol levels and improvement of glucose tolerance. Reduction in weight and regular aerobic exercise also contribute to the reduction of cardiovascular risk.

The treatment of hypertension is one that involves a partnership between patient and physician. Everyone with newly diagnosed moderate hypertension should attempt to control their condition *without* drugs. Cutting down on salt, losing weight, quitting smoking, exercising regularly, and limiting alcohol use will all contribute to improved blood pressure. Some people may be able to avoid antihypertensive medication altogether, though many individuals will still require drug therapies. Doctors no longer follow a "cookbook approach" to the treatment of the hypertensive patient. Every person's situation must be assessed carefully, and the use of medications should be individualized to take into consideration a patient's other illnesses (if any), risk factors, and lifestyle.

There has been much discussion regarding the side effects of blood pressure medication. However, because of the variety of medications now available, there is no need to tolerate side effects that interfere with quality of life.

This book thoroughly covers the diagnosis, evaluation, and treatment of the hypertensive patient. High blood pressure affects so many people that nearly everyone has a family member or a close friend with the condition. The first step, if not the most important step, to the eventual reduction of hypertension, and the related incidence of heart attack and stroke, is a widespread patient education program. *If It Runs in Your Family: Hypertension* is a big step in that direction.

RANDALL M. ZUSMAN, M.D., *Director*
Division of Hypertension and Vascular Medicine
Medical Services, Massachusetts General Hospital
Harvard Medical School
Boston, Massachusetts

1

What It Means to Be at Risk

Chances are you're reading this book because someone in your family has been diagnosed with hypertension, more commonly known as high blood pressure. Or perhaps someone you love, your mother or brother, was one of the 2 million people struck by heart attack or stroke this year because their blood pressure was out of control. Maybe you've even had one or two high blood pressure readings yourself.

If so, you're not alone. Today, an estimated 60 million Americans have high blood pressure, making it one of the nation's most widespread health problems. It is also one of our most serious: Hypertension is the leading risk factor for heart attack and stroke, two of the three leading causes of death in the United States (lung cancer is first).

Are you at risk of developing hypertension and suf-

fering from its effects? If you are at risk, is there anything you can do to prevent it? Take courage: you are
already one big step ahead of the game. Just by being
aware of the importance of blood pressure to your present and future health, you have reduced your chances
of suffering from hypertension and its effects.

Hypertension has long been known as the "silent
killer," because it often has no symptoms until the cardiovascular system is already damaged. Despite the
multitude of warnings sounded by the media about the
importance of preventing or arresting hypertension, literally millions of people still suffer the disease without
being aware of it. A disease is any destructive process
that affects part or all of the body. As you will learn,
hypertension is a destructive process that can damage
specific organs of the body and cause disability and
death.

The good news is that—in most cases—*high blood
pressure may be easily managed.* If you know your risks
of developing the disease, you can make changes in your
diet, exercise, and other personal habits that will help
you avoid the problem. And by preventing hypertension, you automatically reduce your risk of succumbing
to a heart attack, stroke, or kidney disease. The following quiz can help you assess your risk.

Your Hypertension Self-Test

Answer yes or no to the following questions.

Uncontrollable Risk Factors (discussed in chapter 2)

1. Do either or both of your parents have high blood pressure? _____
2. Have any of your siblings been diagnosed with hypertension? _____
3. Have you ever had a high blood pressure reading? _____
4. Are you male? _____
5. Are you over age fifty-five? _____
6. Are you African-American? _____

Controllable Risk Factors (discussed in chapter 3)

7. Are you more than 15 percent overweight?

   _____
8. Do you ingest more than 2 grams of sodium per day? _____
9. Do you exercise less than three times per week?

   _____
10. Do you react to stressful situations with hostility or anger? _____
11. Do you drink more than 2 ounces of alcohol per day? _____

Concomitant Factors (discussed in chapter 3)

12. Do you smoke? _____
13. Do you have diabetes mellitus? _____
14. Do you have high cholesterol (more than 200 milligrams per deciliter)? _____

How many questions did you answer yes to? Every time you answered in the affirmative, your chances for developing hypertension increased. In other words, the risk factors of hypertension are cumulative: If one of your parents has high blood pressure and you're overweight, for instance, you have a greater chance of developing hypertension than if you had a family history of high blood pressure and were of normal weight.

If you answered yes to just one or two questions, you have a relatively low risk of eventually developing high blood pressure. If you answered yes to three to five of the questions, your risk is still moderately low, but may indicate some trouble areas in your diet or lifestyle. If you answered yes to more than five to seven of the questions, on the other hand, you run a moderate to high risk. Eight or nine yeses puts you in a high risk category. More than nine and you are at very high risk.

This test is not meant to frighten you, but rather to help you analyze your risk factors. Just because you have a moderate or even very high risk of hypertension does not mean that you will necessarily suffer from the disease. It simply indicates that you are *more likely* to develop high blood pressure than someone with low risk. This book will help you understand the problem and show you ways to reduce your risks in order to help keep your cardiovascular system healthy and help you live a longer and more active life.

What Is Hypertension?

Just 100 years ago no one, even those in the medical community, knew much about the blood pressure system. Doctors neither measured blood pressure nor understood its relationship to stroke, heart attack, kidney failure, or other medical conditions. It was not until the last twenty or thirty years that the importance of blood pressure was recognized. Blood pressure is defined as the rate and force at which your heart and vessels move blood through the body.

Today, we know that blood pressure is critical to the entire cardiovascular system. If your blood flows through the arteries and veins at too high a pressure, stress is placed on the walls of the heart and blood vessels. This high pressure damages the cardiovascular system in a number of related ways.

The most common damaging result of high blood pressure is the promotion of atherosclerosis or hardening of the arteries. It begins in our teens and progresses in all of us at varying rates and in varying locations. Atherosclerosis builds up like rust on the inside of a pipe and at the same time thickens the blood vessel wall itself and makes it less elastic. As the material builds up on the inside of the blood vessel, the body tries to smooth this over with small blood clots. These little blood clots may break off and go downstream or small pieces of the hardening-of-the-artery material may break off and go downstream. Either of these events, or the complete closing off of the blood vessel itself, can deny portions of affected organs the necessary blood. If the blood is denied to the heart it is called a heart attack. If the brain is deprived of blood it is called a stroke. Gangrene of the leg can develop if the leg is affected in this manner.

The process of hardening of the arteries is promoted by hypertension, smoking, diabetes, and elevated blood fats. The hypertension itself is promoted by excessive salt intake and genetic factors. In addition, smoking and diabetes not only affect high blood pressure but also stimulate the hardening-of-the-artery process directly. As the vessels narrow, the heart and blood vessels must work harder to pump the blood. This also raises blood pressure, adding to the cycle. Drugs can be employed to lessen the hypertension and to diminish the effects of circulating high levels of blood fat. When individuals stop smoking, the body is able to slow down the damaging process and in some instances stop it altogether. Surgery under specific circumstances can be performed to open up, repair, or clean out the damaged blood vessels. Catheters and small balloons have also been used.

High blood pressure can also cause the thin-walled arteries that feed the brain to rupture, causing a stroke in the form of cerebral hemorrhage. Over time, it can weaken the pumping ability of the heart, resulting in heart failure. High blood pressure may eventually damage the eyes and the kidneys by rupturing the vessels that feed them.

What causes blood pressure to become elevated? In most cases, no specific cause can be determined. As we'll explore further in chapter 4, the regulation of blood pressure involves every system in the body: in addition to your heart and blood vessels, your hormones, kidneys, and nervous system are all intricately involved in establishing and maintaining the rate at which your blood is distributed to your bodily tissues and organs. Which of these systems malfunctions to cause hypertension varies from individual to individual and is almost impossible to sort out. When the specific cause cannot be determined the condition is known as *essential hypertension.** Essential hypertension affects between 90 and 95 percent of the hypertensive population.

There are some cases—rare to be sure—when the cause of hypertension can be traced to a specific organ defect or disease. Known as *secondary hypertension,* this condition usually reverses itself once the primary cause is corrected (more about secondary hypertension in chapter 4). Again, however, this condition is quite uncommon, affecting far less than 10 percent of the hypertensive population.

Who are the more than 54 million people who suffer from essential hypertension? Contrary to popular myth, you don't need to be an overworked, highly stressed

---

*Many of the medical terms used in this book are defined in the glossary.

executive to have high blood pressure. Although the term *hypertension* implies stress and anxiety, these emotional factors play a relatively small role in the disease process. The truth is, there is no such thing as a typical hypertensive patient. Hypertension affects people from all social and economic strata, children as well as the elderly, women as well as men, and people of all racial backgrounds. Statistics collected on the incidence of hypertension indicate that there are groups of people who appear to be more susceptible to the disease than others.

What Is a Risk Factor?

Although the cause of essential hypertension is unknown, a number of *risk factors* related to it have been identified. Risk factors are those conditions and habits associated with an increased likelihood of developing a disease. By examining the risk factors for developing hypertension, we are able to identify certain sectors of the population who are *more likely* (although certainly not doomed) to have high blood pressure.

If you look at the box on page 9, you'll see that the risk factors for developing hypertension have been divided into three categories: *Uncontrollable* risk factors are those that are impossible for you to change, including family history, age, gender, and race. *Controllable* risk factors are those things that can be altered, if you choose to make changes in your environment or lifestyle, including diet and exercise habits. For this reason, they are also often referred to as *environmental* risk fac-

---

Risk Factors for Hypertension

Uncontrollable:
- Heredity.
- Age.
- Gender.
- Race.

Controllable:
- Obesity.
- Lack of exercise.
- Stress.
- High salt intake.
- Cigarette smoking.

Concomitant Factors:
- High cholesterol.
- Diabetes.

---

tors. This category also includes smoking and salt intake.

The third category of risk factors for hypertension are labeled *concomitant factors*. Certain conditions, namely high cholesterol and diabetes, are known to coexist with hypertension in many people—and together, they form a deadly combination. A person with high cholesterol *and* hypertension *and* diabetes has a much higher risk of other cardiovascular disease than if any of those conditions are suffered in isolation.

Do not overly concern yourself with category assignments of risk factors. In many ways, they are arbitrary and often overlap. One example is obesity. Although listed as a controllable factor, obesity is known to run in families (uncontrollable). It also is a major risk factor for diabetes and high cholesterol levels (concomitant). Many people believe that heavy drinking, also a controllable risk factor known to cause hypertension in some cases, may also have a genetic component (uncontrollable). High cholesterol and diabetes are also known to run in families, but each of them, in some cases, can be prevented or controlled by diet and exercise. So too can hypertension itself.

What are some of the uncontrollable risk factors associated with hypertension? Many scientists believe that it is possible for an individual to inherit a *genetic predisposition* to hypertension. In other words, along with other traits like eye color and height, your parents may have passed on to you certain characteristics that cause high blood pressure, such as a tendency to retain salt. As you will discover in chapter 2, the genetic link between hypertension is not yet fully understood, but scientists believe that if one of your parents has high blood pressure, you run twice the risk of experiencing the same problem as someone who has no such genetic component.

One clue as to whether you may have inherited a tendency toward high blood pressure is if you have had any high blood pressure readings—even if your blood pressure is normal most of the time. Most people who develop high blood pressure do so between the ages of twenty-five and fifty. Often, the readings are at first normal, then they fluctuate. This is called *labile high blood pressure*.

Labile hypertension is dangerous for two reasons. First, it indicates you may be at risk for full-blown hypertension in the future. Second, the sharp rises in blood pressure—from normal or below normal to very high—within a short period of time may be even more dangerous than sustained high blood pressure that has risen slowly over time. If you have had occasional high blood pressure readings, your risk of hypertension is greater than someone who has not.

Another uncontrollable risk factor is *age*. Although high blood pressure can occur at any age, the majority of patients with high blood pressure are men and women over the age of fifty-five. One study conducted in 1985 showed that more than 50 percent of people over fifty-five years of age were hypertensive. For many years, high blood pressure was considered an almost inevitable side effect of the aging process itself.

It is true that as you get older, more and more physiological changes that affect blood pressure and the health of the circulatory system will take place. Often the artery walls have been damaged by the decades they have worked to pump blood through the circulatory system—even at normal pressure levels. Atherosclerosis (hardening of the arteries) has most likely advanced, and other related diseases like diabetes and kidney disease will have progressed as well.

Until the age of about fifty-five, men generally suffer more hypertension and other cardiovascular diseases than women. Therefore, for people under fifty-five, *gender* should also be considered an uncontrollable risk factor. If you are a young male, you are more likely to have high blood pressure than a female your same age. It is unclear exactly why this is true, but researchers believe that the female hormones estrogen and progesterone play an important role in protecting women from the ravages of atherosclerosis, a contributing factor in the development of hypertension. When women pass the age of menopause, however, the picture begins to change. As female hormone levels decrease, the incidence of high blood pressure in women catches up and even exceeds that of men.

For reasons not yet fully understood, *race* is a factor you should consider when considering your risks for developing hypertension. In general, African-Americans have a one-third higher rate of hypertension than Caucasians. And urban blacks, those who live in major cities, have twice the rate of hypertension and four times the hypertension-induced morbidity (death) rate than a similar white population.

Scientists are still studying why this disparity between African-Americans and Caucasians should be so profound. One theory postulates that many African-Americans may have abnormal levels of renin, a hormone that works to decrease blood pressure. Another explanation may be that some African-Americans are especially salt sensitive: their kidneys are more likely to retain salt and water, which raises blood pressure.

What we do know is that there is no proven correlation between race itself and hypertension stroke. According to studies reported by the Cleveland Clinic, black Africans, for instance, do not suffer the same high rates of hypertension as African-Americans.[†] It is thought that, just as for Caucasian Americans, the generally high-fat, high-salt diets of African-Americans probably cause the majority of hypertension. They may also inherit a predisposition that makes them more sensitive to these dietary factors.

Genetics, age, gender, and race are all aspects of our lives we, of course, cannot control. If you have a family history of hypertension, you do run a higher risk of developing the disease than someone who does not. And if you are African-American, you may be more susceptible to high blood pressure than some Caucasians. However—and this is a *big* however—these factors can almost always be offset by controlling certain diet, exercise, and personal habits that are known to influence the development of the disease.

Risk Factors You Can Control

Since 1972, when the U.S. government first mounted its all-out campaign to alert the nation to the dangers of hypertension, there has been a 50 percent decline in the national stroke mortality rate and about a 40 percent decline in heart disease.[‡] In part, this remarkable ac-

[†]J. V. Warren and G. J. Subak-Sharpe, *Managing Hypertension* (New York: Doubleday & Co., Inc., 1986), 20.
[‡]"The 1988 Report of the Joint National Committee on Detection, Evaluation, and Treatment of High Blood Pressure," *Archives of Internal Medicine* 148 (1988): 1023–1027.

complishment is related to the improvement in both diagnosing and treating hypertension. Some of the most remarkable advances in medicine during the 1970s and 1980s involved the development of safe and effective antihypertension drugs to treat the millions of people with hypertension.

But drugs are only part of the story. More important, a fundamental shift has taken place from treating an existing disease to preventing the disease from ever developing. Both society and the medical profession have participated in this effort. More people than ever are aware that how they live their lives—what they eat, if they smoke, how much stress they have, and how much they exercise—has a profound effect on their present and future health. To cite just one example of the difference this awareness has made, a recent Gallup poll estimates that the number of people who exercise on a regular basis has more than doubled since the early 1960s.

This nationwide trend toward healthier lifestyles is great news for both current hypertensives and those who want to reduce risks of developing the disease. Reducing the controllable (or environmental) risk factors of hypertension will involve the very same diet and exercise modifications everyone—at risk or not—should take to heart: stopping smoking, maintaining a healthy weight, eating less sodium, exercising more often and more vigorously, drinking alcohol moderately or abstaining, and reducing the amount of everyday stress.

Not only will these modifications reduce your chances of developing hypertension but they also will

address many other major concerns related to cardiovascular health. Without doubt, hypertension itself is a
major health problem. But hypertension often does not
work alone. Instead, many people at risk for high blood
pressure have other diseases or conditions that may further compromise the health of their cardiovascular
system.

As we will discuss in more depth in chapter 3, these
concomitant factors, including smoking, high cholesterol, and diabetes, are intricately linked to high blood
pressure. The combination of these and other factors in
relationship to cardiovascular disease is also known as
the *multiple risk phenomenon*. Research on the multiple
risk phenomenon proves that the risk of heart attack
and stroke rises dramatically with every risk factor (hypertension, high cholesterol, cigarette smoking, and diabetes, among others). Because living longer and in
better health is your ultimate goal, a discussion on preventing hypertension and its effects would not be complete without taking these concomitant, multiple risk
factors into consideration.

A Lifelong Commitment

Look again at the results of "Your Hypertension Self-
Test." Are you at risk for developing high blood pressure? If so, know that there are ways for you and your
family to reduce those risks considerably. Even uncontrollable risk factors can be balanced by proper diet and
exercise. Today, we know that with proper habits the

risks of developing hypertension can be greatly diminished.

Maintaining your blood pressure at a safe and normal level is a lifelong proposition. There are no quick fixes here, no vaccines or surgical procedures that will keep you from ever developing hypertension. Instead, it takes a commitment from you to start eating right, exercising regularly, and finding ways to deal appropriately with the stress of modern life. That commitment should be shared by other members of your family—your mate, your children, and your parents. In addition, friends and colleagues are very important. Lifestyle changes such as diet, exercise, and quitting smoking can obviously be affected and influenced by people at work and outside the home. After reading this book, you will be able to share with them your knowledge of the risks—and the ways to reduce those risks—of hypertension.

Questions and Answers

Q: I have a family history of both high blood pressure and heart attacks. Which is more important for me to do: lose weight or stop smoking?

A: That's a difficult question to answer. The link between obesity and hypertension is more conclusively drawn than the one between smoking and hypertension. We know that, in general, the more you weigh, the higher your blood pressure. High blood pressure is implicated in most cases of heart attacks and strokes. However, the overall effect on your cardiovascular health from cigarette smoking is, in most cases, far more damaging than the rise in blood pressure in relation to excess weight. As we'll discuss in chapter 5, unless you're severely obese (more than 20 percent of your ideal weight), your cigarette smoking poses a greater health risk to you than your excess poundage.

Q: So far, my blood pressure is normal, but the disease runs in my family. Should I worry about my children's blood pressure?

A: You are never too young to have hypertension and it's never too soon to begin a lifelong plan to avoid it. If you have a family history of hypertension (see chapter 2 to evaluate your own genetic background) and have children, it is important to monitor their blood pressure carefully. By instilling proper diet and exercise habits in your children from a very young age, you could help them—as well as yourself—avoid high blood pressure and its side effects.

2

The Genetic Factors

Does hypertension run in your family? Are you older than fifty-five? Are you African-American? If so, you may be more susceptible than others to the development of hypertension. As discussed in chapter 1, these factors are called uncontrollable risk factors, uncontrollable because, obviously, you can do nothing about your ancestry, your age, or your race. However, by being aware that one or more of these factors put you at risk, you are in a position to avoid the ravages of this silent, symptomless disease before major damage is done. Consider the following case history.*

A Case History

One night Charles, a fifty-two-year-old salesman, his wife, Rebecca, and a twenty-five-year-old daughter, An-

*All names and identifying information of individuals mentioned in this case history have been changed to protect their privacy.

gela, were watching television. Charles was energetically discussing a news story with his daughter when he suddenly began feeling short of breath. This was accompanied by pain in his left chest that went up to his jaw. He could not catch his breath and described a sensation of something heavy on his chest. At the same time, he began perspiring and told his wife and daughter that he was feeling very anxious.

Frightened, he asked his wife and daughter to telephone for the paramedics, thinking he was having a heart attack or a stroke. The ambulance arrived, the paramedics started an intravenous line, gave Charles some medication, and took an electrocardiogram en route to the hospital.

After a series of tests were performed in the next few days, it became clear that Charles had coronary artery disease. This was explained to him as a lack of blood supply to the heart. He had experienced angina when his heart increased its rate of beating during his emotional discussions. The tests at the hospital showed that he did not have a heart attack but they did show some mild narrowing of the blood vessels in his heart from atherosclerosis. One of the main blood vessels to his heart was narrowed by atherosclerosis or plaque. This had been seen on a coronary angiogram, a special dye study of the blood vessels of his heart. In addition to this, some spasm or intermittent narrowing of the blood vessels accounted for the decreased blood flow to his heart muscle. His chest pain was due to an inability of the heart itself to get enough blood during a period of increased activity. A drug was prescribed for Charles that would reduce the spasm in the blood vessels and would increase the blood flow to his heart.

With his medical emergency over, Charles was forced to take a look at his entire medical condition: What caused his angina and how could he avoid having even more serious cardiovascular events?

Charles was shocked to find out that not only did he have high blood pressure (about 165/100 millimeters of mercury) but he also had a cholesterol level in the danger zone, approaching 230 milligrams per deciliter. Although Charles still considered himself to be in great physical shape, his "little spare tire" actually weighed some 20 pounds, making him about 15 percent above his ideal weight.

Charles's physician, Dr. Clark, sent him home with some stern admonishments. To avoid another cardiovascular event, Charles had to get his blood pressure and other medical problems under control. Dr. Clark was prepared to issue a number of prescriptions for medications, but Charles, not being much of a pill taker, asked his doctor if it was possible to treat his blood pressure and high cholesterol without using drugs.

Although Dr. Clark insisted that Charles take medication to lower his blood pressure on a short-term basis, Charles was assured that if he made several lifestyle changes the drug would be gradually withdrawn. Charles and his wife met with a dietician that very afternoon and were happy to learn that if he carefully followed a sensible diet, exercise plan, and stress reduction plan, he would *probably* be able to control his major health problems. He resolved to put the plan into effect immediately.

Although the family was thrilled that Charles would be all right—at least in the short term—Angela had a few special concerns.

Angela had heard that hypertension and the risk for heart attack and stroke ran in families. She wanted to know what factors in her father's family background and his own medical history caused his blood pressure to rise so precipitously. And what would this genetic and medical information mean to Angela and her siblings? Because Charles had high blood pressure, did it mean that she and her brother and sister were doomed to develop hypertension, too?

If one of your grandparents, parents, or other close relatives has been diagnosed with high blood pressure or has suffered a serious cardiovascular event like the one Charles had, you are probably asking yourself, "Will I develop hypertension, too?" No simple answer to that question exists. However, this section will help you understand the issues involved in the genetic connections.

The Genetic Connection

Every one of the cells in your body, of which there are literally millions, contain genetic material you've inherited from your parents. Deoxyribonucleic acid, commonly known as DNA, is the basic genetic component. Approximately 10,000 DNA pairs comprise a gene. A number of genes together, sequenced in a certain order, make up a genetic code. It is this coded information that determines, to a large degree, how each cell develops and functions.

The largest genetic structure in the cell is called the chromosome. Each chromosome is made up of long strands of DNA chains. Every one of your cells contains forty-six chromosomes, twenty-three inherited from your mother and twenty-three inherited from your father. And all of this material and the information it contains exists in a tiny dot of fluid, bound by a very thin membrane, known as the cell. When the cells of each individual begin the process of differentiation—dividing into liver cells, brain cells, and so forth—early in the development of the embryo, the genetic material, encoded in the chromosomes, is reproduced and passed along in each new cell.

It is through this remarkable organization that you have inherited many of your unique physical characteristics, intellectual capabilities, and personality traits from your parents. It is also how you may have inherited a predisposition to hypertension. It is important to understand that with hypertension there is no genetic certainty that you will inherit the disorder.

All human disease—including hypertension—can be considered to result from an interaction between an individual's unique genetic makeup and the circumstances under which he or she lives: environmental conditions that include personal habits, such as diet and exercise patterns and stress levels, as well as exposure to pollution and other toxins. The genetic differences between human beings, including those in the same family, determine not only such things as hair color and IQ, they also determine the ability of each individual to meet environmental conditions, including those that produce disease.

In certain disorders, the genetic component is so strong that nothing within an individual's power will alter the course of the disease. These diseases, such as hemophilia and cystic fibrosis, are relatively rare. They fall into the two categories of genetic diseases known as chromosomal disorders and simply inherited disorders. Chromosomal disorders are caused by the lack, excess, or abnormal arrangement of one or more chromosomes. Simply inherited disorders are caused by a single gene that has mutated (changed abnormally).

Most common adult diseases, such as hypertension and heart disease, however, are known as multifactorial disorders. They are caused by an interaction of multiple genes and multiple environmental and lifestyle factors. In a multifactorial disease, there are many different genes responsible for causing the chronic condition; geneticists have identified at least seventeen genes that participate in just one aspect of coronary heart disease, for example.*

In addition, many of those genes express themselves differently depending on the circumstances. If a person who has inherited a tendency to retain sodium—often an important factor in hypertension—never eats salt, he

*R. Henig, "High-Tech Fortunetelling," *The New York Times Magazine,* March 18, 1990, 20.

or she will probably not develop high blood pressure. In other words, despite a genetic predisposition to the disease, environmental factors, including lifestyle and personal habits, will outweigh the genetic component in most individuals.

As far as geneticists can determine, *first-degree relatives*—parents, siblings, and children—have about a 10 percent chance of experiencing exactly the same multifactorial disease as the affected individual. Although that may seem like a fairly low percentage, it represents *twice* the risk of someone who has no history of hypertension in his or her family. According to Dr. Kenneth Cooper,[†] that means that

> if one of your parents or one of your siblings has hypertension, you run twice the risk of experiencing the same problem as someone who has no such genetic component.

Your risk of developing hypertension is even greater if your fraternal or identical twin has been diagnosed with the disease.

The Genogram

Not everyone with a family history of a multifactorial disease will necessarily inherit it, and more important, not everyone who inherits such a disorder is doomed to

[†]K. H. Cooper, *Overcoming Hypertension* (New York: Bantam Books, 1990), 55.

suffer from it. But because there are often few—if any—overt symptoms of hypertension, it's important to assess your own genetic predisposition in time to prevent it from damaging your body.

Creating a family genogram, a family tree annotated with medical history, can increase your awareness and provide an understanding of your family's history of disease. Even if you think you know your family history, putting it down on paper can help you establish connections among events that at first glance may seem unrelated.

Start by drawing a family tree that spans at least four generations: yourself, your siblings (if any), your children (if any), your parents, and your grandparents. In preparing the skeleton of your family tree, you may want to use the standard genogram symbols recommended by the Task Force of the North American Primary Care Research Group and described in *Genograms in Family Assessment* by Monica McGoldrick and Randy Gerson (W. W. Norton & Co., 1985). Or you can invent any symbols you like in creating your own family tree, as long as you make sure to distinguish between male and female and living and deceased members of your family. The standard genogram symbols are shown at the top of page 27. In addition to these basic symbols, you may want to draw a double line around yourself to distinguish yourself from the rest of your family.

Because research shows that people with hypertensive first-degree relatives are at the greatest risk for developing hypertension themselves, that is where you should start your search for genetic links. You can begin

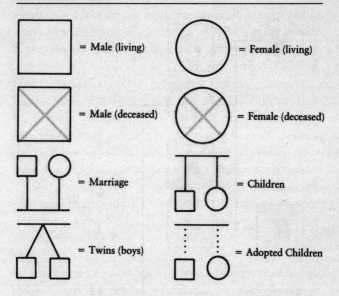

to get an idea of your own inherited risk for hypertension by tracing the disease along the branches of your family tree.

First, fill in everyone's name and year of birth, as well as the year of death for those deceased. When you have finished drawing the skeleton of your family tree, you will have a diagram that resembles Figure 1.

Once you have this skeleton, you can begin adding specific notes that will help you trace your family history of hypertension. Be as thorough as you can in filling in what you and other relatives know about the occurrence of hypertension and other related diseases in your family. Unfortunately, until about twenty years ago, hypertension was even more of a silent killer than it is today. Those who died of strokes, heart attacks,

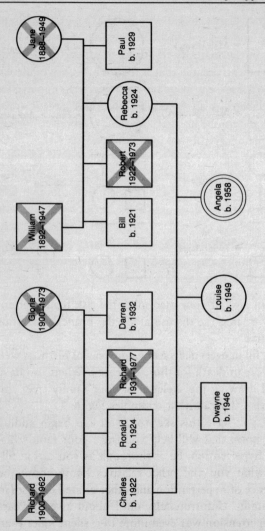

Figure 1.   Angela's Genogram—Skeleton.

and kidney disease might very well have had high blood pressure and never known it. Because hypertension is present in the majority of stroke and heart attack patients, you can assume that if there's a history of stroke and heart disease in your family, hypertension played a part. Diabetes is an especially important genetic trait. Try and determine its approximate age of onset for any family members affected by this disease as well.

In addition to specific medical information, make sure you investigate another aspect of your family history: the controllable or environmental factors that add to the risk of hypertension. Cigarette smoking, high salt intake, obesity, and heavy drinking are almost as likely to be passed along as genetic diseases. And they are often far more important to you in determining your chances of developing hypertension.

To give you an idea how a genogram might look, I've included Angela's efforts in deriving her family medical tree. Figure 1 is the skeleton of Angela's family tree. Figure 2 was developed after Angela learned more about the other genetic factors responsible for hypertension. You, too, will find yourself able to fill in more and more information as you read this book. In order to get some of this information, you may need to do a little digging. Ask your relatives if they can fill in any of the gaps. Perhaps your mother knows that her father and brother both had high blood pressure, a fact you might not have known. Don't get stuck on tracking down every last detail. Just get your best impression of the risk factors among your relatives.

Let's take a look at what Angela found out from her

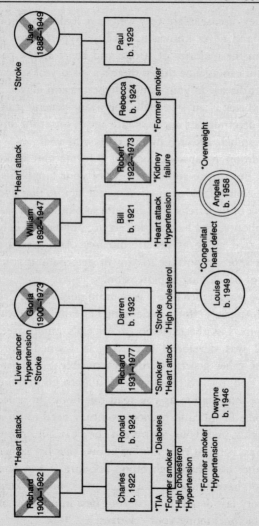

Figure 2.   Angela's Genogram—Completed.

genogram. Although Angela's mother did not have hypertension, Angela knew it was important to check that side of the family as well as her father's. What she found was disturbing: her maternal grandmother had two strokes related to high blood pressure and her grandfather had died suddenly of a heart attack. Among Angela's mother's brothers, kidney disease had killed one brother and high blood pressure led to a heart attack in another.

The paternal side of Angela's family is also important: both high blood pressure and diabetes are found. Her paternal grandfather died of a heart attack. It is not known whether or not he had high blood pressure. Her grandmother died of cancer, but before she died, high blood pressure had caused a stroke. One of her uncles had two minor strokes related to atherosclerosis. Another uncle died of a heart attack quite young. One of the sons developed diabetes—another hypertension cohort—when he reached his fifties.

What does this family history mean to Angela? It means that she and her siblings have to monitor their blood pressures very carefully. They know that from heredity alone they run about twice the risk of developing hypertension as someone who does not have such a problematic family history.

Angela and her family also noted that high cholesterol and diabetes, listed as concomitant factors in this text, also run in their family. In about 25 percent of all diabetes cases, there is a family history of hypertension.

Your Genetic Risks

When you examine your family tree, what signs do you see that indicate you might be genetically predisposed to hypertension? Have members of your immediate family been diagnosed with hypertension? Who has suffered a stroke or a heart attack?

Armed with the information you've received from constructing your own family genogram, you can work on eliminating or reducing those risk factors that *are* controllable—some of which you may have learned from your parents, like eating salty foods, gaining weight, or smoking, which will be covered in depth in chapters 3 and 5. And make sure that you are not the only one to benefit from this information. If hypertension is present in a family, it is important that all family members have their risk profiles assessed. If you have children, educate them and teach them the rules of prevention outlined in this book. Help them understand their genogram and its implications for their health.

Questions and Answers

Q: I'm adopted and don't know anything about my biologic parents or their medical histories. Is there any way for me to figure out if I've inherited a risk for hypertension?

A: From a purely genetic standpoint, no, unless the agency that handled your adoption has kept medical files on your parents. However, because many of the risk factors for cardiovascular disease are more *environmental* than genetic, you may be able to assess at least part of your risk by examing the dietary habits of your adoptive family—excess salt and dietary cholesterol are known to contribute to the risk of developing hypertension. Cholesterol will be discussed in detail in chapter 5.

Q: Neither of my parents are hypertensive and no one in my family has suffered a stroke or heart attack. Do I still need to worry about these diseases?

A: Hypertension and the cardiovascular events such as stroke, heart attack, and kidney disease that result from it are multifactorial diseases. The genetic component, therefore, is a small part of the overall hypertension picture.

3

The Environmental Factors

Could it be that simply growing up in the United States is a risk factor of hypertension? In general, Americans eat too much fat, salt, and dietary cholesterol, and don't get enough exercise. In addition, our hectic lifestyles promote stress. We smoke too much, drink too much alcohol, and ingest too much caffeine. The result of these poor diet and exercise habits is that we have among the highest levels of hypertension, strokes, and heart attacks in the world.

On the other hand, the word about these lifestyle pitfalls has reached across the country. More and more of us are eating healthier foods, exercising on a regular basis, and striving to find a balance in our lives between stress and relaxation. Health consciousness is taking hold. A recent Gallup poll showed that weight loss, for instance, is no longer the predominant motivation for a change in diet: Preventing disease would motivate nearly 50 percent of the people polled to change their eating habits.

The Gallup Survey of
Food and Eating Habits 1989*

If you were considering making a change in your eating habits, what would be your main reason for change?

To prevent heart disease 27%
To lose weight 26%
To feel better 25%
To treat a specific health problem 15%
To prevent cancer 5%
Don't know 2%

*Based on a telephone survey of 1,016 adults from January 16 to 27, 1989. Sampling error is plus or minus 4 percentage points. This poll was conducted by The Gallup Organization, Inc., for *Cooking Light* and *Hippocrates* magazines. Reprinted with permission.

How about you? Do you consider yourself a healthy, fit American? Or do you have one or two (or more) bad habits that may put you at higher risk of developing hypertension and other cardiovascular disease?

To assess your environmental risks, put a check mark next to each condition or habit in the following list that relates to your lifestyle.

Controllable Risk Factor Checklist

1. _____ I am overweight.
2. _____ I consume an excess of salt (more than 2 grams per day).
3. _____ I exercise (running, aerobic dance, swimming, cycling, brisk walking, or other aerobic activity) less than three times a week.
4. _____ I react to stressful situations with anger and/or hostility.
5. _____ I regularly drink more than 2 ounces of alcohol per day.
6. _____ I smoke.
7. _____ I am diabetic.
8. _____ My blood cholesterol level is above 200 milliliters per deciliter.
9. _____ I take birth control pills.

Remember, the more environmental risk factors you checked off, the greater risk of high blood pressure you run—especially if you carry a genetic predisposition to the disease. Don't be discouraged. Even if you've checked off several of these negative influences, you can have a positive impact on all of these risk factors. Some, such as diabetes, can be controlled with drugs, but most can be controlled by you.

To find out how your dietary or exercise habits may be putting you at risk of developing hypertension, read

the sections of this chapter that apply to you. You
should read them all. Even if you're thin now, for instance, you should know what putting on just a few
pounds might mean to you in the future.

Am I Overweight?

The Facts. The statistics on the dangers of obesity are
overwhelming: The famous Framingham Heart Study,
in which 5,000 patients from Framingham, Massachusetts, were monitored for cardiovascular disease over
four decades, showed that patients who were 20 percent
or more over their ideal weight were *eight times more
likely to become hypertensive* than their thin peers. The
same study showed that a 10 percent increase in weight
is accompanied by an increase of 6.5 points in blood
pressure; as weight increased, so did blood pressure levels. See Tables 2 and 3 on pages 84 and 85 to see if
you are overweight.

The Connection. Blood pressure is determined by
two things: the volume of blood that the heart pushes
into circulation and the resistance to flow created by
the tension of the muscles within the walls of the arteries. The fat stored in your body is no different from any
other body tissue: it needs to be fed by the bloodstream.
To supply extra fatty tissue with oxygen and other nutrients, the body must increase the total amount of fluid
in the bloodstream. This causes the walls of the arteries
to expand. Because of this increased stretch, there is
increased tension pressing inward on the bloodstream

contained within the arteries. Thus the heart pumps a larger load through arteries that exert an increased resistance to flow.

You can see now how even a gain of 10 pounds would put an increased burden on your heart and blood vessels; for each pound of excess weight, your heart is forced to pump blood through an additional several hundred miles of blood vessels a day. In addition to this direct correlation between weight and blood pressure, someone who is overweight should consider several other related issues. Overweight people tend to eat too much fat and cholesterol, which contributes to atherosclerosis. They also tend to exercise less. Obesity and diabetes are also twin threats: most diabetics are overweight, and many overweight individuals will develop diabetes.

Reduce Your Risks. According to most medical specialists, losing weight, if you are overweight, is the single most reliable method of preventing the development of, or lowering existing, high blood pressure. One Framingham researcher remarked, "If everyone [in the study] had maintained his or her ideal weight there would have been 25 percent fewer heart attacks at any age in either sex."

Keep in mind that it's never too early to worry about your weight and its relationship to your health. Obese children who remain overweight are more likely to develop high blood pressure, and at an earlier age, than their normal weight peers. If your weight is normal now, work hard to keep it that way. If you are overweight, try to lose weight (see chapter 5 for more information).

Do I Eat an Excess of Salt?

The Facts. Most research shows that approximately 30 percent of people who develop high blood pressure are salt sensitive. Their high blood pressure is partly related to the amount of sodium (one of salt's main ingredients) they consume. Studies also show that if someone is genetically predisposed to hypertension, excess sodium in the diet can be the trigger for the progression of high blood pressure. See chapter 5 if you think your diet may be too high in sodium.

The Connection. The actual physiological need for sodium may be as low as 220 milligrams a day, but most Americans consume more than ten times that amount, at least 2,500 milligrams (2.5 grams) each day. This puts an incredible strain on the kidneys, which play a crucial role in the maintenance of blood pressure in the body.

The kidneys regulate the blood pressure by retaining sodium, thereby increasing the volume and pressure of the blood, or excreting sodium and fluid, thereby decreasing blood volume and pressure. If you consume too much salt and your kidneys are unable to excrete it, the level of fluids in your body will rise. This causes blood pressure to rise, because the vessels and heart must work that much harder to circulate the extra fluid.

Exactly why this occurs in some people and not others is as yet unknown.

Reduce Your Risk. Ask your doctor how salt may affect your high blood pressure. If one of your relatives is known to be a salt-sensitive hypertensive, there's a good chance that you, too, run the risk of developing the disease if you consume an excess of sodium. It was once thought that everyone who had high blood pressure had to put away the saltshakers and give up canned soups forever, but chapter 5 provides more up-to-date dietary tips and information.

Do I Lead a Sedentary Life?

The Facts. One study conducted by the Cooper Clinic in Dallas followed more than 6,000 adults who had normal blood pressure. Four years later, the clinic found that those who engaged in regular exercise had a 34 percent lower risk of developing hypertension.[*] Although there is no conclusive proof that lack of exercise causes high blood pressure or that increased physical activity can prevent it, there is a statistical link between exercise and a healthy circulatory system.

The Connection. When the body is exercising, blood volume to and from the heart rises to about 25 quarts per minute. This extra work strengthens the heart mus-

[*]S. N. Blair et al., "Physical Fitness and the Incidence of Hypertension in Healthy Normotensive Men and Women," Journal of the American Medical Association 252 (1984): 487–490.

cle; the stronger it is, the easier it is for the heart to meet the body's need for oxygen. The heart works more efficiently. Continued and consistent exercise also results in the dilation or expansion of the blood vessels. Both of these actions lower blood pressure.

Vigorous exercise also helps to reduce cholesterol levels and helps to prevent or control diabetes by aiding the metabolism of carbohydrates and other sugars. In addition, exercise often leads to weight loss, because the more calories you burn up, the less will be stored as fat. As we have seen, obesity plays a major role in the development of hypertension. Another benefit of exercise is that most people find that it releases tension and stress.

Reduce Your Risk. With your doctor's permission, begin a regular program that has you exercising thirty to forty-five minutes per session, three or more times a week. In chapter 5, we will discuss in detail why exercise is important to your cardiovascular health and how to choose the right exercise program for you.

Do I React to Stress with Hostility?

The Facts. In 1984, an article in *The Wall Street Journal* revealed the results of a remarkable, twenty-five-year study. A group of men were given a standardized personality test that measured, among other things, hostility. Twenty-five years later, it was found that the death rate of the men with the higher hostility scores was 4.2 times greater than that of men who had low scores.† There is general agreement that stress and the way we deal with it has a direct impact on our health, including our blood pressure.

However, statistically measuring that impact and the effect of methods developed to diminish it (such as biofeedback and meditation) is a difficult task. One reason is that stress and the way one reacts to it are almost impossible to measure objectively. In addition, as is true for many aspects of hypertension, stress rarely exists as the *sole* risk factor in any given person. In chapter 5, you'll read more about the theories of stress and hypertension, including the well-known theory of Type A (harried, obsessive, and angry) and Type B (confident, calm, and friendly) personalities.

One thing is certain: Although stress may play a role in the development of hypertension, it is not the only cause of the disease. Indeed, many hypertensive patients are calm, easygoing, and enjoy a relatively tension-free lifestyle.

The Connection. The connection between stress and blood pressure seems to be the ways in which, and the levels to which, certain people produce the "fight or flight" stress hormones, norepinephrine and epinephrine. These hormones work to stimulate the heart and blood vessels to raise the blood pressure in reaction to danger or stress. Usually, the elevated arterial pressure returns to normal a short while after the stressful situation has been alleviated. However, if an individual is

†L. W. Gibbons and N. F. Gordon, *The Cooper Clinic Cardiac Rehabilitation Program* (New York: Simon & Schuster, 1990), 275.

unable to cope with stress on a continuing basis, hypertension can theoretically result.

Reduce Your Risk. Many people find that relaxation methods, which include biofeedback and meditation among others, will significantly lower blood pressure if practiced regularly. (Biofeedback is a relaxation method that uses electronic instruments to measure and reveal to a patient bodily activities, such as heart rate, respiration, blood pressure, and so forth, of which there is usually no awareness. Using electrodes taped to the chest, for example, a patient can "see" his or her heartbeat on an electronic monitor. When the patient sees a green light, the heart rate is low; a red light indicates it is high. The patient then attempts to either speed up or slow his or her heart rate by consciously "urging" the heart to do so.) One study, conducted in London during the early 1980s, showed that hypertensive patients practicing biofeedback techniques reduced their blood pressures by more than twenty points *systolic* and ten points *diastolic* (more on what these figures mean in chapter 4).[‡]

Do I Drink Too Much Alcohol?

The Facts. Studies have shown that heavy drinkers—those who consume 3 to 5 ounces or more of alcohol

[‡]C. Patel and M. Marmot, "Can General Practitioners Use Training in Relaxation and Management of Stress to Reduce Mild Hypertension?" *British Medical Journal* 296 (1988): 21–24.

a day—have a higher incidence of hypertension than those who drink moderately or who abstain. Dr. Kenneth Cooper, in his book *Overcoming Hypertension,* cites research connecting alcohol consumption and hypertension in a very graphic way: 80 percent of hypertensive patients entering an alcohol rehabilitation program end up with normal blood pressure within thirty to sixty days after they stop drinking.

The Connection. Most of us think of alcohol as a relaxant; we have a drink or two to unwind. Indeed, the initial effects of alcohol often are relaxing, both mentally and physically. Our heart rate is slowed and our blood vessels are dilated, meaning that our blood pressure is lowered while the alcohol is in our system.

The trouble starts when the effects of alcohol wear off. Our bodies often overcompensate for the relaxation effect, pushing our heart and blood pressure rate up quickly, often above our normal rate. Individuals who drink on a regular basis, or who drink excessively, have blood pressure that remains elevated over a long period of time. As we know, this increases the likelihood of permanent cardiovascular disease.

A limit of 2 ounces of alcohol or less per day probably has little permanent effect on blood pressure. Some studies, although still controversial, have shown that moderate drinking provides some protection against heart attacks and strokes.

Reduce Your Risk. If you don't drink, don't start. If you do, limit your alcohol intake to 2 ounces or less a day. That translates into one jigger of eighty-proof liquor, one 12-ounce serving of beer, or two 6-ounce glasses of wine.

Can Smoking Affect My Blood Pressure?

The Facts. Smoking tobacco produces a temporary rise in blood pressure, but current research indicates that it does not directly cause sustained hypertension. As Dr. Ray Gifford of the Cleveland Clinic, quoted in *Managing Hypertension* by Jame V. Warren, M.D., wrote, "Cigarette smoking is especially harmful . . . not because it increases hypertension, but because it is an independent risk factor for the same things that hypertension is a risk factor for."* In other words, smoking increases the risk of heart attack and stroke.

The Connection. When you smoke a cigarette, cigar, or pipe, nicotine enters the bloodstream and reaches the brain within six seconds. This occurs whether or not you inhale. Nicotine is a stimulant; when it reaches the brain, it signals the adrenal glands to release the hormones norepinephrine and epinephrine (adrenaline), which increases both the systolic and diastolic blood pressures. Your heart beats faster and pumps more blood, and your arteries work harder to contain this increased pumping action. This, as we know, elevates the blood pressure.

In addition to directly causing an increase in heart

---

*J. V. Warren and G. J. Subak-Sharpe, *Managing Hypertension* (New York: Doubleday & Co., Inc., 1986), 24.

and vessel activity, cigarette smoking also contributes to the buildup of atherosclerosis, hypertension's deadly partner. There are some 4,000 substances identified in cigarette smoke—some highly toxic and carcinogenic (cancer causing).

Reduce Your Risk. Plainly and simply, stop smoking as soon as you can (see chapter 5 for tips).

What If I'm Diabetic?

The Facts. Diabetes mellitus is defined as an inability to metabolize carbohydrates, specifically sugar. A diabetic either does not produce enough insulin, which is the hormone largely responsible for regulating the body's metabolism, or is unable to utilize the insulin properly.

According to statistics compiled by the American Heart Association, approximately 15 percent of hypertensives also have diabetes. Although there is no direct correlation between diabetes and the development of hypertension, diabetes is a definite risk factor for other cardiovascular diseases. In the Framingham Heart Study, 75 percent of the deaths among diabetic men were caused by strokes and heart attacks; for women diabetics, death from cardiovascular disease was 80 percent. About three-fourths of the deaths among diabetic patients are caused by cardiovascular complications.

The Connection. How diabetes promotes cardiovascular disease is unclear, but many researchers think that the abnormally high sugar levels in the bloodstream promote atherosclerosis. In addition, diabetes has damaging effects on the capillaries, the smallest blood vessels that nourish individual cells.

Reduce Your Risk. Like hypertension, diabetes often runs in families. Symptoms of the disease include excessive thirst and frequent urination. If you feel you are at risk for both hypertension and diabetes, it's more important than ever to see your doctor, be tested for both, and learn how you can protect yourself from the complications of these diseases. Often, mild cases of diabetes mellitus can be controlled by diet and exercise. In other cases, drugs are necessary; see your physician.

Do I Have High Serum Cholesterol?

The Facts. Cholesterol is one of a number of fatty substances, called lipids, found in the body. Cholesterol is both consumed in the diet and produced by the body. When too much cholesterol circulates in the bloodstream, atherosclerosis and coronary artery disease often result.

There are two different types of cholesterol, each defined by the type of protein that carries it through the bloodstream. Low-density lipoproteins (LDLs) are known as the "bad cholesterol" because they carry cholesterol into body tissues, including the walls of blood vessels. High-density lipoproteins (HDLs) are known as the "good cholesterol" because they carry cholesterol away from cells and tissues. Many researchers believe that the ratio of the HDL level to the total serum cholesterol level is as important as the total cholesterol level.

The Connection. Cholesterol's relationship to high blood pressure is one of a deadly partner: The two work together to promote atherosclerosis—the damage and weakening of arteries due to the buildup of fat. Scientists believe it often works in the following manner: High blood pressure slowly but steadily wears down blood vessel walls, creating pockets of scar tissue. Then high levels of cholesterol and other fats circulating in the blood collect in those pockets, narrowing the vessels—a condition known as atherosclerosis.

Reduce Your Risk. Have your cholesterol level measured soon. A common myth about high cholesterol is that only overweight people are susceptible. In fact, anyone, especially someone with a family history of high cholesterol, can have the disease. Like hypertension, however, most cases of high cholesterol are controllable by diet and exercise. Limit the amount of fat you consume to about 30 percent of a day's total calories (400 calories or less for those dieting to lose weight) and make sure that just 10 percent of that amount consists of saturated fats (see chapter 5 for more details).

What If I Take Birth Control Pills?

The Facts. The use of oral contraceptives raises blood pressure *slightly* in virtually all women who take them. For some women, however, they cause a dramatic rise in blood pressure, putting those women at increased risk for stroke and heart attack. Like many other facets of hypertension, the risk of using the Pill increases when other risk factors are added into the equation. For example, some studies show that the risk of stroke or heart attack in women who both smoke and take the Pill could be up to ten times that of women who do neither. Other risks which, when combined with the Pill promote hypertension, include age (older than thirty-five), diabetes, and a history of breast or ovarian cancer.

The Connection. There are two types of birth control pills currently in use in the United States. One is called a combination pill. It contains two hormones, progestin and estrogen. The other is called a minipill, which contains progestin only. Both pills work by intervening with normal fluctuations in hormone levels, thereby preventing the egg from maturing and being released into the uterus.

In terms of the risk of hypertension from the Pill, the hormone estrogen appears to be the culprit. Estrogen acts to stimulate the production of a certain natural substance, called *angiotensin II*. Angiotensin II, produced in the kidney, is responsible for setting off a chain reaction ending with the raising of blood pressure (more about angiotensin in chapter 4).

Reduce Your Risk. If you have a family history of hypertension; if you are over thirty-five years of age; or if you smoke, have diabetes, or breast or ovarian cancer, you probably should choose another method of birth control. This is a matter best discussed with your gynecologist.

* * *

Now that you've learned about the risks—genetic, environmental, and concomitant—of developing hypertension, it's time for you to find out about blood pressure itself. How is it measured? How should you evaluate your measurement? What systems in the body control it? And, perhaps most important, how high *is* high blood pressure?

4

What Is Hypertension?

Chances are, if you are concerned enough about your blood pressure to be reading this book, you have probably had your blood pressure taken recently. If you haven't, make an appointment with your physician immediately; a blood pressure exam is one of the easiest and most informative tests in medicine.

As quick and painless as the procedure is, it is one of the most useful diagnostic exams around—if done correctly. As you will see when you read the following sections on how blood pressure is measured, the procedure does have two basic requirements: accurate equipment and a knowledgeable, alert practitioner. For that reason, it is suggested that, at least until you are familiar with your own blood pressure readings and fluctuations, you visit your own physician, rather than an unfamiliar walk-in clinic for your blood pressure exams.

How Blood Pressure Is Measured

To calculate blood pressure, we focus on the two stages of heart and vessel action: (1) the heartbeat, which pumps blood that has collected inside the heart out to the arteries, and (2) the heart at rest, when it is filling with blood and the arteries are pushing the blood throughout the body. The first action is called *systole,* which means the contraction of the heart; the blood pressure is at its highest point during systole. When the heart is at rest, filling with blood, the blood pressure is at its lowest. We call this stage *diastole.*

Blood pressure is measured by an instrument called a sphygmomanometer, invented by the Italian physician Scipione Riva-Rocci in 1898. This instrument allows physicians to calculate how hard the heart is pumping and how much the blood vessels must contract to push the blood along.

The sphygmomanometer is made up of three components: an inflatable cuff, which is attached to a pressure gauge measured in millimeters, and a stethoscope. As air is pumped into the cuff, the pressure is raised within the gauge. The gauge may be a digital readout, a round dial reading, or a vertical column of liquid mercury.

Anyone who's had his or her blood pressure taken will remember the procedure. First, the physician or examiner wraps the cuff snugly around the upper arm and pumps air into it until the cuff is tight enough to keep blood from flowing. The stethoscope is then placed on the arm just below the cuff, and listening carefully, the physician slowly releases the air from the cuff.

What the doctor is listening for is the sound of the first spurt of blood as it passes through the artery; this represents the systolic pressure, the maximum pressure that is required to push the blood from the heart and move it through the arteries. The position of the gauge or of the mercury in the column gives the first number of the blood pressure reading.

The doctor continues to listen to the sound of the blood moving through the vessel as he or she lets more and more air out of the cuff. At the point when the cuff is no longer restricting the blood flow and the doctor hears no sound at all, the diastolic pressure is read. This is the pressure that the arteries exert on the blood while the heart is filling up; it is the pressure in the circulation between heartbeats.

If your blood pressure is 120/80, it means that the first spurt of blood flow through your artery was when the pressure in the cuff pushed the gauge to 120 millimeters. The pressure had fallen to 80 millimeters by the time all external pressure had been removed.

Although a blood pressure exam is simple and completely painless, it's important to realize that it's not always 100 percent accurate. Any of the following could cause you to receive an inaccurate reading, either a false high or false low.

- *Accuracy of the equipment.* One of the most common problems with gaining accurate blood pressure readings involves the equipment itself. A critical element is the cuff, the part of the sphygmomanometer that wraps around your upper arm. If the cuff doesn't fit properly, an inaccurate measurement is likely. The cuff should encircle at least two-thirds of your arm from the elbow to the shoulder. If the cuff is too big, a child-size cuff may be more appropriate. If the cuff is too small, a thigh cuff—originally designed to measure blood pressure in the leg—should be used.

- *Accuracy of the reader.* Good hearing is essential to an accurate blood pressure reading. Should the doctor or examiner be distracted by noise or be hard of hearing, the blood pressure reading could be off by a significant amount. In addition, the stethoscope must provide adequate amplification and the room in which the blood pressure is taken should be quiet. This is especially important when it comes to getting an accurate diastolic measurement; remember, your physician or examiner is listening for the *absence* of sound in this case. Keep in mind that good vision and concentration is also required to watch the blood pressure gauge as it falls.

- *Anxiety.* Are you terrified of going to the doctor? Some people are, and when they have a blood pressure reading taken in the doctor's office it is often within the hypertensive range. Does that mean they are clinically hypertensive? Not necessarily. It may mean that they suffer from what Dr. Kenneth Coo-

---

*K. H. Cooper, *Overcoming Hypertension* (New York: Bantam Books, 1990), 41.

per refers to as the "white coat syndrome."* According to studies, notes Dr. Cooper, the only place this patient's blood pressure is high is in the doctor's office.

What causes this to occur in some individuals is as yet unclear. If you become overly nervous or tense when you visit your physician and have received one or more high readings, you may want to consider learning to take your own blood pressure at home. You will still need to see your doctor to compare results.

- *Your physical condition.* Any number of things could cause your blood pressure to rise for a short period of time, giving you a high blood pressure reading when, in fact, your blood pressure is normal most of the time. Two cups of coffee or a cigarette just before the exam, for instance, can distort your reading.

For all of these reasons, the Joint National Committee on Detection, Evaluation, and Treatment of High Blood Pressure recommends that more than one, and preferably three, separate blood pressure readings be taken during a physical exam and an average reading be calculated.† If you have one averaged reading that's particularly high, your doctor will probably recommend that you come back in a few days or a week to take another reading. If it is normal on that occasion, he or she may want to give you yet another set of readings a

† "The 1988 Report of the Joint National Committee on Detection, Evaluation, and Treatment of Blood Pressure," *Archives of Internal Medicine* 148 (1988):1023–1027.

week or two after that. The average of these three averaged readings should give you an accurate measure of
your blood pressure.

If your averaged reading is normal, can you then ignore the one high reading? Not necessarily. You may
be one of a category of people referred to as *labile hypertensives,* first discussed in chapter 2. Someone with
labile hypertension has normal blood pressure most of
the time, but occasionally experiences sharp rises in
pressure. Labile hypertension is a cause for concern for
two reasons. First, it may indicate a predisposition for
the development of true hypertension, especially if you
have a family history of the disease. Second, depending
on how drastically your blood pressure shoots up, your
blood vessels may be damaged by the high, although
occasional, rises in pressure. Discuss this matter with
your physician, especially if high blood pressure runs in
your family.

Evaluating Your Blood Pressure Reading

Perhaps you've been told by your doctor that your average blood pressure reading is in the normal range, say
135/85. Does such a "normal" reading mean that your
blood pressure is at a safe and healthy level? Probably.
Even doctors still disagree over what constitutes normal
and high blood pressure.

Our blood pressure is never constant. It fluctuates
when we exercise, eat, sleep, argue, and relax. Literally
hundreds of factors—external and internal—affect the
level of arterial pressure. Having hypertension, how-

Table 1.
Classifications of Blood Pressure Measurements

Class	Reading (in milliliters of mercury)
Systolic	
Normal	140 or lower
Borderline	141–159
Severe	160 or higher
Diastolic	
Normal	85 or lower
High-normal	86–89
Mild	90–114
Severe	115 or higher

ever, means that our heart and vessels are working too hard all the time, even when we're calm and at rest. Hypertension must be brought under control, by diet and exercise or through the use of antihypertensive drugs, or severe damage to the cardiovascular system will occur.

How high is *too* high? Although general categories have been established (see Table 1), the truth is that no exact dividing line exists between normal and high blood pressure. Most agree, however, that a reading of 120/80 is absolutely normal and anything between 110/70 and 140/90 is within the normal *range*. However, someone with normal blood pressure who has a family history of hypertension and/or is overweight, salt sensitive, or sedentary may not stay within the normal range for very long.

Borderline hypertension is any reading between 140/90 and 160/104. Most of the 60 million people with high blood pressure in the United States fall into this category. Like those with normal pressure but at high risk, most borderline hypertensives can treat their disease with diet, salt restriction, and weight control.

A reading of 160/104 to 190/115 indicates *moderate hypertension*. The heart, vessels, and kidneys are at greater risk of damage. Depending on the general health of the individual, changes in diet and exercise habits may be enough to bring blood pressure back into the normal range. If concomitant risk factors, such as diabetes or high cholesterol, are involved or if the pressure is on the high-moderate side, a combination of antihypertensive drugs and dietary modifications may be prescribed.

Any reading above 190/115 is considered *severe hypertension*. This condition requires immediate treatment with powerful antihypertensive drugs to prevent a medical crisis. Once the blood pressure falls within a moderate range, the physician may gradually decrease drug therapy, as long as the patient continues to comply with the recommended lifestyle modifications.

There are two other categories of high blood pressure: *isolated systolic* and *isolated diastolic* hypertension. As their names imply, these conditions occur when just one aspect of your blood pressure system is abnormal. It was once thought that the systolic reading (the first number) rose naturally as a kind of side effect of the aging process. In fact, an old rule of thumb was that your systolic reading was normal if it was 100 plus your age. That meant that a man of 40 has normal systolic pressure at 140, while someone 70 years of age fell within the normal range at 170. Doctors believed that the diastolic (the second number) pressure was a better indicator of true high blood pressure. Only if the diastolic reading was higher than 95 or 100 was the older patient considered to be hypertensive.

Recently, that thinking has changed. One study, referred to as MRFIT (for Multiple Risk Factor Intervention Trial), found that an isolated high systolic—*not* diastolic—reading was the major factor in deaths from cardiovascular disease in the more than 3,000 men who were tested. Today, we know that both measurements are equally important in assessing health. The higher either reading is, the greater the health risks. If both readings are high, the effects on the circulatory system will be even more pronounced.

Although these categories give you a general idea how to evaluate blood pressure readings, judging your own personal reading is another matter. Let us say, as we did at the beginning of this section, that you were given a clean bill of blood pressure health with a reading of 135/85. But does that mean that your heart and vessels are being damaged?

That's a difficult question to answer with any certainty. Blood pressure, as we've seen, is a relative matter. Most studies show that the higher the blood pressure, the greater the risks of disease—*even if they fall within the normal range.* Generally speaking, someone with a blood pressure of 110/70 runs fewer cardiovascular health risks than someone with a blood pressure of 120/80. In turn, the person with a 120/80 reading may fare better in the long run than the person whose pressure is measured at 135/85.

What is the bottom line then? For most people, the lower the blood pressure, the better, as long as it falls within the normal range. A reading of 110/70 is considered by most physicians to be the lowest safe blood pressure in most individuals. Anything below that is called *hypotension,* or low blood pressure. Unlike hypertension, hypotension has a number of warning signs including dizziness, weakness, and lethargy. (Ironically, many patients suffer from hypotension after taking antihypertension medication; see chapter 6 for more details.) Your own "correct" blood pressure is determined by your weight, height, age, and other individual physical characteristics.

Although conclusive symptoms of hypertension are rare, there are a number of clues that might let you know that your blood pressure is out of the healthy range. If you should experience any of the following, it may be an indication that your blood pressure is out of control:

- Frequent headaches.
- Chronic fatigue or weakness in certain muscles in the arms and legs.
- Bouts of dizziness.
- Shortness of breath.
- Blurred vision or changes in the field of vision.

Unfortunately, many of these symptoms are inconclusive—they could mean you have high blood pressure or they may reflect perfectly normal fluctuations in blood pressure, body temperature, and other bodily functions. It is also important to remember that most people who have high blood pressure have no symptoms. The symptoms above are uncommon. Most of the time there are no symptoms until some complication of hypertension such as heart attack or stroke occurs.

The Blood Pressure System

To say that the human body works like an efficient machine is to make a vast understatement. No machine carries out as many complicated interrelated tasks; the amount and complexity of functions required to keep us thinking and learning, moving and growing, and seeing and feeling is truly astounding. Using a complex internal network, our various organ systems constantly attempt to work together in the perfect harmony we know as health.

Perhaps most amazing of all is that the majority of these functions are performed silently, unconsciously. We are usually quite oblivious to our inner workings: We read books, play tennis, digest food, and make love completely unaware of the number of hormones, enzymes, muscles, and nerves required to keep us on the go.

Often when we focus on one specific disease, we tend to lose sight of this most important aspect of human physiology: no one system of the body is separate from the others. Although hypertension is a disease of the circulation, for instance, we must go far beyond the vessel walls to understand the dynamics of the blood pressure system and how it gets out of control. We must examine many different organ systems in addition to the circulatory system: the hormones our body produces, the ways in which our kidneys function, and how the nervous system coordinates our bodily functions are the keys to understanding the development of high blood pressure.

Inside the Circulatory System

More than 70 percent of the human body is made up of fluids and about 5 percent of our total body weight consists of the fluid we know as blood. In order to live, each cell of the body must have a steady supply of oxygen and other nutrients brought to it by the bloodstream, which then carries away from the cell carbon dioxide and waste matter. The human circulatory system, which transports these nutrients and wastes, consists of two main components: the blood itself and the vessels that carry the fluid.

At the center of this system is a mass of specialized muscle tissue known as the heart. About the size of your fist, this amazing organ beats an average of 72 times a minute, 100,000 times a day, pumping your blood through about 70,000 miles of blood vessels at the rate of more than 1 gallon a minute. Essentially a sophisticated pump, the heart rhythmically contracts to force the blood out through the vessels and then back to the heart. The average adult has about 11 pints of blood, which the heart pumps through the body. Every time the heart beats, it sends 2 to 3 ounces of blood from its pumping chamber, the left ventricle, into the body's largest artery, the aorta. From the aorta branches the large arteries that supply blood to the head, internal organs, the arms, and the legs. These large arteries branch into smaller and smaller vessels, the smallest of which are arterioles and capillaries, which bring the blood into every cell in the body. On the way back to the heart, the blood travels through veins and their smaller subset, venules. It takes less than a minute for a drop of blood to travel through the body, and as noted above, there are about 70,000 miles of blood vessels in the average human body.

All vessel walls are made up of muscle tissue that can expand and contract to push the blood along its route, but the arteries, and especially the arterioles, have the greatest portion of *smooth muscle* in their walls. Veins, on the other hand, do not contain nearly as much muscle tissue and, therefore, have little effect on the blood pressure. It is the contraction and relaxation of the muscle tissue in the arteries that regulates the flow of blood to each organ system; it is the action of the arteries and arterioles that is measured in a blood pressure reading.

Blood pressure, then, can be defined as a combination of the heart's action (systole) and the force of the contractions necessary to push the blood through the body (diastole). But how does the heart know how much blood to pump? And what tells the vessel walls how hard to contract or dilate?

The Body's Thermostat

Just as other bodily functions require cooperation between systems, so too does the regulation of blood pressure. While the force required to keep blood moving through the body originates in the heart and vessels, two other organs—the kidneys and the sympathetic nervous system—work together to control the blood pressure.

The role of the circulatory system in this process is critical: the harder the heart pumps, the more blood is forced into the arteries. The more blood in the arteries, the higher the pressure on the arterial walls. To keep the blood flowing in the appropriate amounts, the arteries contract to keep the blood flow steady; the harder they must contract, the higher the blood pressure.

The kidneys, a pair of bean-shaped organs that lie at the base of the abdominal cavity, are another essential part of blood pressure control. By eliminating waste products and water from our bodies through the production of urine, the kidneys regulate the level of fluid in the body, including the blood. The kidneys determine the amount of fluid in our bodies by either retaining salt and water or by eliminating salt and water. This affects blood pressure in two ways. First, it raises the amount of fluid in the body, forcing the heart and the vessels to work harder simply to move the fluid through the body.

Second, when the kidney retains fluid, this excess fluid collects in the tissues throughout the body and stretches them. When there is too much fluid in the tissues, the tissues can become stiff, making it more difficult for the blood to leave the arteries to nourish the cells. The arteries must contract harder to push the blood out into the tissues, and again, the blood pressure goes up.

The sympathetic nervous system, the part of the nervous system that controls unconscious functions such as blood pressure and respiration, is responsible for sending messages to and from the heart, arteries, and kidneys. Arterial muscle tissue, for instance, is supplied with what are called vasomotor nerves, which regulate the expansion and contraction of the vessel walls.

As a result of a variety of factors, the supply of blood required by the cells normally changes, and the vasomotor nerves work to accommodate these changes. When we exercise, for instance, our voluntary muscles need more oxygen; our arteries will expand to bring more blood into the area and the heart beats faster. When we eat, more blood is then carried to our intestines so that digestion can begin. Blood flow to these areas is controlled by involuntary muscles and the autonomic nervous system.

Working like the thermostat that automatically regulates the heat in our homes, other groups of sympathetic nerve cells, called baroreceptors, also help to control the body's blood pressure. If one part of the blood pressure system is set too high or too low, the other parts of the system—after being "alerted" by the nervous system—will work together to bring the blood pressure back to normal. One of the most important baroreceptors, the carotid sinus, is a pressure-sensitive cavity located in the wall of the major artery that carries blood to the brain. This important artery is called the carotid artery.

The carotid sinus makes sure that there is enough blood under the proper pressure getting to the brain. If the blood supply is threatened in any way, it will send out messages to other parts of the body to raise the blood pressure. In other words, a fall in blood pressure brings about a corresponding drop in carotid artery pressure. The carotid sinus then sends messages to the arteries to constrict and the heart to beat harder and faster.

Hormones and Blood Pressure Regulation

An essential link between the sympathetic nervous system and the heart and vessels is the endocrine system, the part of our anatomy that is responsible for producing a special class of hormones. These chemicals in essence "deliver" the nervous system messages by stimulating the reactions in the body to those messages. Hormones produced by the adrenal medulla, an endocrine gland within the kidneys, play a particularly important role in controlling blood pressure.

When the sympathetic nervous system senses danger or stress, for instance, it signals the adrenal medulla to release its two primary hormones, epinephrine and norepinephrine. These are also known as the fight or flight stress hormones. Epinephrine makes the heart beat faster, and norepinephrine causes the blood vessels to constrict; both of these actions, as we've seen, cause an elevation in blood pressure.

Other hormones work within the kidneys to regulate the amount of salt and water in the body. One of these substances is called aldosterone; when the kidney secretes aldosterone, more salt and water is retained by the kidneys. Accordingly, blood pressure is raised as the heart and vessels work to pump this increased amount of fluid throughout the body.

Another hormone secreted by the kidney is thought to be a key mechanism in the blood pressure system. Called renin, this hormone works in combination with another hormone, angiotensin. Whenever the kidney senses the need to raise the blood pressure, it secretes renin into the bloodstream, setting off a chain of events that ends with angiotensin reacting with yet another hormone, angiotensin II, that then causes the walls of the arteries to constrict, which raises the blood pressure.

In addition, angiotensin II stimulates the release of aldosterone which, you'll remember, causes the kidneys to retain salt and water. The renin-angiotensin-aldosterone system is not completely understood as yet, but research has shown that it is a crucial factor in the control of normal blood pressure and the development of high blood pressure.

What Causes Hypertension?

In essence, when someone has high blood pressure, it means that one or more of the following three actions are taking place: (1) messages from the sympathetic nervous system force the heart to pump harder and faster, (2) the nervous system "tells" the kidneys to retain more salt and water, or (3) the arteries and arterioles receive the message to constrict. Precisely what makes the sympathetic nervous system—the body's thermostat—set the blood pressure system too high is a question that continues to be a focus of considerable research.

Essential Hypertension. In most cases, no one cause of elevated blood pressure can be diagnosed. As noted in chapter 1, about 90 percent of all hypertensives are said to have *essential* hypertension—no one cause for it can be identified. The main difficulty in pinpointing the source of the trouble is the extremely interrelated nature of the systems that control blood pressure. The vascular, hormonal, renal, and autonomic nervous systems are all involved, working in complex unity to regulate blood flow throughout the body. Often, a patient at risk of developing essential hypertension may have more than one abnormality in more than one of those systems.

Secondary Hypertension. In approximately 10 percent of hypertension cases, a specific cause can be identified for the elevated arterial pressure. This is known as secondary hypertension. Hypertension in these cases is caused by certain diseases that are identifiable and are most often curable with drugs or surgery.

Renal hypertension is one type of secondary hypertension. It occurs when one of the mechanisms for sodium and fluid retention within the kidney becomes damaged or when the kidney secretes too much of the hormone renin, which causes constriction of the arteries and encourages sodium and fluid retention. Kidney disease, including infections, tumors, or obstruction of the arteries, is often the cause of secondary hypertension, especially in children. Many of these conditions can be alleviated with surgery to remove a tumor or remove an obstruction; after surgery, the blood pressure either returns to a normal level or is more easily controlled.

Disturbances within the endocrine system may also cause secondary hypertension. In rare cases, tumors form in the adrenal gland, which cause it to secrete increased amounts of the hormones epinephrine and norepinephrine. These hormones act to stimulate the heart and constrict the blood vessels. Another rare hormonal disease is primary aldosteronism, when an excess amount of the hormone aldosterone causes a depletion of potassium and an increase of sodium in the bloodstream.

A congenital blood vessel disease, coarctation of the aorta, is a serious defect, resulting in severe hypertension. In these cases the main vessel leading away from the heart, the aorta, is partially closed off by a constriction of its wall. The treatment of coarctation of the aorta is surgical; without surgery the risks for hypertension, stroke, and heart attack are enormous, especially in children.

In many instances, the causes and effects of hypertension are one and the same. Like the proverbial chicken and egg story, it is difficult to figure out which came first in the development of hypertension. Did high blood pressure cause kidney disease or was there some kidney disease first, creating hypertension? Many physicians

are finding it difficult to separate completely essential
hypertension from secondary hypertension, unless there
is a specific organ defect, such as an adrenal tumor.

If the hypertension goes untreated, however, a fatal
and rapidly progressive form can result. About 1 percent of all hypertensive patients develop what is called
malignant hypertension. It is a serious, often fatal, form
of the disease. Paralysis, *convulsions,* and *coma,* resulting from a significantly increased flow of blood to the
brain, are some of the results of malignant hypertension.

In general the health and welfare of your circulatory
system is the single most important factor in keeping
your brain and your heart alive and well. You must
keep your blood pressure at a normal level, and this is
a lifelong proposition. As discussed in chapter 3, it
means watching what you eat and drink, exercising regularly, and most important, keeping careful track of
your blood pressure by having regular physical exams.
It is far easier to lower slightly elevated blood pressure
than to recover from a stroke or heart attack caused by
undiagnosed high blood pressure.

Taking Your Own Blood Pressure

If you have a family history of hypertension and want
to keep a close watch over your blood pressure, you
may want to consider monitoring your own blood pressure at home. This way, you can see exactly what effect
your controllable risk factors have on your blood pres-

sure levels as you reduce and modify them (see chapter 5). If you have already been diagnosed with borderline or moderate hypertension, you will be able to keep more careful watch on your condition at home. In either case, you may be able to save yourself at least a few trips to the doctor's office.

Most people can easily learn to take their own blood pressure. All it takes is an accurate sphygmomanometer and some practice. The first step is to choose which home monitoring device to purchase. Because there are so many different makes and models on the market, many people consult *Consumer Reports* or their physicians for advice on which model is best for their needs. You should also check with your physician before making the purchase. Accuracy, ease of use, and cost vary considerably among models.

In general, there are two different types of monitoring devices. The least expensive and, luckily, the most accurate is the *manual mercury manometer*. At about $15 to $45, this machine is quite reliable when used appropriately, but it can be tricky for the novice. It involves listening through a stethoscope and reading a gauge. *Electronic mercury manometers* tend to be less accurate (they are very sensitive and may give false readings unless used with extreme care—directions as to where to place the cuff and how still to hold the arm must be precisely followed), more expensive (from $45 to $90), but are far easier to use. They operate on batteries and automatically give the pressure readings on a digital display panel.

If you decide to purchase an electronic device, be

aware that not only are they less accurate to begin with but they are also more fragile. If they are dropped or bounced around, they may become even more inaccurate or break altogether. Check the readings you get from an electronic manometer against a mercury device at frequent intervals.

There are also a variety of fingertip blood pressure devices available. Although apparently simple, they are often inaccurate and the blood pressure reading unreliable.

In general, the same rules apply to taking your own blood pressure as were described at the beginning of this chapter for office exams—the equipment should be accurate and the environment quiet. You should take several readings, especially when you first start out, and compare your measurements with those you've received at your doctor's office. If you need help with your equipment or in evaluating your readings, make sure to discuss it with your doctor. Below is an easy, step-by-step procedure for taking your own blood pressure.

1. Choose a quiet, calm room where you won't be interrupted; being able to hear clearly is essential.
2. Sit down. Because most information on treatment is taken from seated measurements, it is best to sit down while you take your reading.
3. There should be a table next to the chair; when you rest your forearm flat on the table, your upper arm should be at about the same level as your heart.

4. Use your fingertips to feel the pulse in the crook of your elbow; this is the pulse of the brachial artery, and it is from this artery that you will measure your blood pressure.

5. Slip on the blood pressure cuff and close it tightly around your arm above the elbow.

6. Place the stethoscope in your ears.

7. Put the pressure gauge where you can easily see it.

8. Inflate the cuff until the mercury in the pressure gauge measures about 30 millimeters above your expected systolic pressure (if your last blood pressure reading at the doctor's office was 130, inflate the cuff until the gauge measures 160 millimeters).

9. You should not hear anything through the stethoscope at this point; now, very slowly release the pressure in the cuff using the release knob on the bulb.

10. As soon as you hear a beat through the stethoscope, record the number indicated on the pressure gauge; this represents the systolic pressure.

11. Continue to let air out of the cuff; you will continue to hear a thumping noise as blood rushes past the cuff, although the sound will get softer and softer as the pressure against the artery is released. When you no longer hear a sound, record the measure indicated on the pressure gauge; this represents the diastolic pressure.

12. If you want to make sure your measurement is accurate, repeat the reading.

It may help your physician to also know what your pulse rate was, and the time and date of the reading. Your pulse rate is the number of times your heart beats per minute (explained further in chapter 5).

No matter what your blood pressure measurement is now, it is never too early or too late to take an active role in controlling it. Start to reduce your risk of developing hypertension or lower your blood pressure if it is already too high by eliminating as many of the controllable risk factors as you can. If you are overweight, ask your doctor to create a weight-loss program. If you consume too much sodium, substitute other seasonings for the salt in your diet. Restrict your fat intake if your cholesterol level is high. If you're stressed out and sitting at a desk all day, get out of the office, get some exercise, and try to relax. And if you smoke, stop.

We all know how very difficult it is to break habits, but in the next chapter, you will find out exactly why such changes are vital to the health of your circulatory system. You will also learn some helpful hints that should get you on the road to maintaining and improving your health.

5

Preventing Hypertension

Now that you've evaluated your genetic and environmental risks and learned about the science of blood pressure measurement and evaluation, you can take the next step: finding safe and effective ways to reduce your risk of hypertension. Where should you begin?

Look at the "Controllable Risk Factor Checklist" on page 37. Are you overweight? Do you eat too much salt? Have you been unable to make exercise a part of your daily life? Do you smoke? You are not alone. Millions of Americans run these same risks of hypertension. The good news is that millions of others have recognized the problem and organized a program to control their risk factors and improve their health. You can do it too.

Taking Preventive Action Now

Every day new admonitions about our dietary and life-style habits are sounded by various health organizations and the advice can be confusing. It is difficult to keep it all straight. Is there such a thing as "good" choles-terol? Is running harmful or healthy? How much fiber is enough? To eat oat bran or not to eat oat bran?

Although this book cannot answer all these questions or guarantee you a long and healthy life, by the time you finish reading this chapter you will probably realize that there are some major changes you can begin to make to-day that will considerably reduce your risk of developing high blood pressure and improve your health.

And, in very basic ways, these changes are related. Eat-ing less fat will usually result in weight loss, reducing the risk of hypertension that accompanies excess weight. Ex-ercising also contributes to weight loss and often inspires people to quit smoking. Despite its trendiness, then, the term "healthier lifestyle" describes quite succinctly the best advice for reducing your risk for developing high blood pressure. This healthier lifestyle also helps lower your blood pressure if you already have hypertension.

This chapter is divided into four sections: The first discusses the way weight control and a proper diet can help to prevent or reduce high blood pressure. The ap-proach is threefold. First, with help from the American Heart Association, we will explore what a healthy diet entails for all of us, overweight or not, who are at risk for hypertension. Then it addresses three separate, but related, dietary problems: too many calories, too much salt, and too much cholesterol and other fats. You will find out how each of those problems can lead to or exacerbate hypertension and how to improve your eating habits to reduce this risk.

The second section covers exercise. Only slightly more than 50 percent of all Americans exercise more than once a week, and only 30 percent of us exercise enough to derive any real cardiovascular benefits. Yet, the *Journal of the American Medical Association* has advised that "previously sedentary people can safely bring moderately high blood pressure under control without drugs if they are willing to exercise vigorously for 50 minutes three or four times a week."* Additional studies show that even just 20 to 30 minutes of moderate excercises performed on a regular basis os enough to lower risks. The benefits of exercise to someone who does not yet have high blood pressure are clear. Adding regular, vigorous exercise to your routine could add years to your life.

The third section will explore the link between stress and hypertension. Is it possible that our internal thermostats get set too high because of the ways in which we psychologically handle day-to-day aggravations and environmental challenges? You will see that there are methods—short of moving to an island paradise—that may help you reduce this stress and, therefore, prevent hypertension.

---

*J. Brody, As quoted in "Exercise Rated As Good As Drugs for Blood Pressure," *The New York Times,* May 19, 1990, Section A, 32.

Finally, although stopping smoking will not prevent you from developing high blood pressure directly, it is the single most important controllable risk factor for cardiovascular disease. No book about the health of the cardiovascular system would be complete without a section on cigarette smoking and the damage it does to the heart, lungs, and blood vessels. In this section, you will not only learn about the effects of smoking but you'll also find some tips that may help you to stop.

If one section in this chapter interests you more than another, feel free to skip to that section. Be aware that there are literally hundreds of books about diet programs, exercise plans, and stress reduction and there are thousands of different theories about each of these lifestyle components. Because the scope of these subjects is beyond the limits of this chapter, consult the resources in chapter 8, in your local bookstore and public library, and ask your doctor for more guidance. Reading to improve your health and well-being is a good way to learn what nondrug therapy will best help you reduce *your* risk for hypertension.

Weight Control and Healthy Eating

It really is true: You are what you eat. What you consume today could very well increase or decrease your chances of developing hypertension in the future.

The variety and amount of food you eat affects your chances for cardiovascular disease in three basic ways:

- If you consume too many calories, you will gain weight; obesity and high blood pressure are often deadly partners.
- If you consume too much sodium, studies indicate that you run the risk of elevating your blood pressure.
- If you consume too much fat and cholesterol, you are more apt to develop atherosclerosis, which is hypertension's most deadly cohort.

Although these three dietary factors may appear to be quite separate—someone who eats too much salt may not be overweight, for instance, and vice versa—a sensible eating plan, like the one devised by the American Heart Association and followed by many reputable weight loss organizations such as Weight Watchers, addresses all three problems at the same time.

The American Heart Association's Dietary Guidelines for Healthy American Adults

According to the American Heart Association, a typical modern American gets more than 40 percent of his or her calories from fat, about 20 percent from complex carbohydrates (vegetables, grains, and fibers), 20 percent from sugar, and the other 20 percent from protein. Changing the above percentages will go a long way in helping you to lose weight and protecting you against cerebrovascular disease.

In order to achieve and maintain cardiovascular and cerebrovascular health, the following dietary guidelines should be followed:

1. Total daily fat intake should be less than 30 percent of calories; of this percentage, only 10 percent should consist of saturated fats.
2. Daily cholesterol intake should be less than 100 milligrams per 1,000 calories; not to exceed 300 milligrams per day.
3. Protein intake should add up to 15 percent of each day's calories.
4. Carbohydrate intake should constitute 50 to 55 percent or more of daily calorie intake, with emphasis on increased complex carbohydrates such as grains and legumes.
5. Sodium intake should be reduced to approximately 3 grams per day.
6. Alcohol intake should be limited to 15 percent of total calories and not exceed 50 milliliters of ethanol (pure alcohol) per day (about 2 ounces of liquor or two glasses of beer).
7. Total calories should be sufficient to maintain proper body weight.
8. A wide variety of foods—fruit, vegetables, dairy products, protein (meat, chicken, fish, and nuts), and carbohydrates (bread, pasta, and grains)—should be consumed (see pages 100–101 for more information).

Obesity and Hypertension

Although it often seems that Americans are preoccupied with body image and although some people who diet do not in fact need to lose weight, there is no doubt that obesity remains America's number one nutritional problem. According to the American Heart Association, more than 150 million Americans are overweight. Of that number, approximately 25 million are considered obese; that is, they are 20 percent or more above their ideal weight for their height, build, and sex (see Tables 2 and 3). One article published in the *American Journal of Public Health* rather graphically estimated that altogether adult Americans carry an excess of 2.3 billion pounds of fat.

Obesity is a leading factor in many of our chronic diseases, hypertension included. The Framingham Heart Study showed that the level of blood pressure rises in direct correlation to weight. According to Framingham researchers, a 10 percent increase in weight is accompanied by an increase of 6.5 points in blood pressure.[†] Obese people also have higher rates of stroke, heart attack, atherosclerosis, diabetes, and kidney disorders than their thinner counterparts. Needless to say, those who are significantly overweight are more likely to die at a younger age than their thinner peers.

Why some people become overweight and others re-

[†] T. R. Dawber *The Framingham Study: The Epidemiology of Atherosclerotic Disease* (Cambridge, Mass: Harvard University Press, 1980).

Table 2.
Desired Weights of Men
Aged Twenty-five and Over

Height	Small Frame	Medium Frame	Large Frame
5'2"	128–134	131–141	138–150
5'3"	130–136	133–143	140–153
5'4"	132–138	135–145	142–156
5'5"	134–140	137–148	144–160
5'6"	136–142	139–151	146–164
5'7"	138–145	142–154	149–168
5'8"	140–148	145–157	152–172
5'9"	142–151	148–160	155–176
5'10"	144–154	151–163	158–180
5'11"	146–157	154–166	161–184
6'0"	149–160	157–170	164–188
6'1"	152–164	160–174	168–192
6'2"	155–168	164–178	172–197
6'3"	158–172	167–182	176–202
6'4"	162–176	171–187	181–207

Courtesy of Metropolitan Life Insurance Company.

main slim, even while appearing to eat the same amounts of food, is not yet completely understood. Age, genetics, metabolism, and a host of other factors all contribute to an individual's propensity to gain or lose weight. Like hypertension, obesity is a multifactorial disorder that goes hand-in-hand with other diseases—especially diabetes and atherosclerosis—that also run in

Table 3.
Desired Weights of Women
Aged Twenty-five and Over*

Height	Small Frame	Medium Frame	Large Frame
4'10"	102–111	109–121	118–131
4'11"	103–113	111–123	120–134
5'0"	104–115	113–126	122–137
5'1"	106–118	115–129	125–140
5'2"	108–121	118–132	128–143
5'3"	111–124	121–135	131–147
5'4"	114–127	124–138	134–151
5'5"	117–130	127–141	137–155
5'6"	120–133	130–144	140–159
5'7"	123–136	133–147	143–163
5'8"	126–139	136–150	146–167
5'9"	129–142	139–153	149–170
5'10"	132–145	142–156	152–173
5'11"	135–148	145–159	155–176
6'0"	138–151	148–162	158–179

Courtesy of Metropolitan Life Insurance Company.
*Women between the ages of eighteen and twenty-five should subtract 1 pound for each year under age twenty-five.

families and that also predispose someone to hypertension.

Although no one knows exactly why or how obesity causes hypertension, it has been proven in several studies that losing weight is one of the safest and surest ways to lower high blood pressure. A study conducted in Israel in the late 1970s (reported in the *New England*

Journal of Medicine in 1976), for instance, showed that 79 out of 81 patients who lost an average of 20 pounds decreased their blood pressure by an average of 30 millimeters of mercury (the substance used in the manual mercury manometers) systolic and 20 millimeters of mercury diastolic.

Unfortunately, as many of us know, losing weight and keeping it off is difficult.

Why Do You Eat?

Eating, like all other human behaviors, is controlled not by the digestive system alone, but with the cooperation of many different organ systems throughout the body, including, most important, the autonomic nervous system. The hypothalamus, a part of the forebrain, controls much of our eating behavior.

Within the hypothalamus are two separate control organs. The feeding center part of the hypothalamus signals to the cerebral cortex, that part of our brain responsible for initiating voluntary activity, that we are hungry and to begin eating. The other part of the hypothalamus, the satiety center, lets the feeding center know when we are no longer hungry. The hypothalamus then signals the cerebral cortex that we are full and to stop eating.

Technically, these activities take place because other parts of our bodies signal to the hypothalamus that we need nutrition or that we have enough food. The satiety center, for instance, may be activated by the increases of glucose and/or insulin that are secreted when carbohydrates are being digested. Gastric distension, caused by the intestines stretching to accommodate ingested food, may also inhibit the eating impulse.

There is also evidence that each of us has a set point of fatty tissue in our bodies, a certain amount of fat cells that is built into our physiological makeup. This level may be inherited. We eat enough to maintain that set point; when we fall below it we feel hungry. How the set point is established or how the hypothalamus senses how much fatty tissue is present in the body is not fully understood. But this theory does explain why it is so difficult for many of us to lose weight—and how very easy it is for such a person to gain weight back after losing.

The regulation of eating behavior is one of the least understood aspects of human physiology, mainly because so many other factors than actual hunger and satiety are involved. If we only ate when we were hungry and only consumed what our bodies needed to survive, the diet-related problems of hypertension, heart disease, and other disorders would be greatly diminished. However, there are so many social and cultural factors involved in eating that treating it as a simple biological process is impossible.

Hunger is, for many overweight people, the last of a long list of reasons to eat: boredom, frustration, stress, depression, excitement, and social exchanges, not to mention that food simply tastes good, are just a few of the non–hunger-related reasons for eating. Add to that list a genetic predisposition to obesity and the stage is set for many of us to grow up with weight problems.

Although some people can eat without gaining weight, it does not necessarily mean that the odds are forever against everyone else. Millions of people have lost weight by learning new eating behaviors. While our shapes and sizes are, to a large degree, predetermined by genetics, there are very few of us who cannot achieve a healthier weight through diet and exercise.

To help you understand why and what you eat, many nutritionists suggest keeping a detailed food diary, writing down every morsel of food you ate and when and *why* you ate. (Were you eating because it was time for a meal and you were hungry? Were you eating because you were at the movies and craved popcorn?) That way, you can not only monitor how many calories you take in and the types of food you consume but also discover some of the reasons *why* you eat what you do. Are you a nighttime muncher of potato chips? Or an eggs-bacon-and-toast-for-breakfast-every-morning person? If you know when you are most likely to overeat, you will be able to find substitutes for that behavior. For instance, some people find the hours right after work but before dinner to be particularly troublesome; for them, choosing that time to exercise may be a good way to keep them away from food until mealtime.

Instead of concentrating only on counting calories, many physicians and dieticians recommend that you educate yourself about proper nutrition in general, taking into consideration your own food preferences and habits when choosing a weight-loss method. The most successful and medically safe ways to lose weight are those that both reduce caloric intake and allow for a healthy variety of food.

Fad diets that promise rapid weight loss and concentrate on eating just a few select foods are dangerous for many reasons. If you only concentrate on losing pounds and not learning proper nutrition, once you go off your diet you will probably fall back into the same kinds of bad eating habits that made you heavy in the first place. This kind of seesaw effect is both dangerous and counterproductive; rapid weight loss puts an extraordinary strain on the cardiovascular system and also changes the body's metabolic rate, lowering the number of calories your body needs to maintain vital functions (and lowering the number of calories you burn when you exercise). That is why people find it difficult to lose weight again after crash dieting.

Sodium and Hypertension

Perhaps no other dietary component has come under as much scrutiny in the study of hypertension as the mineral sodium. Sodium is an essential substance, needed in the body to regulate the amount of water retained by the body. This helps maintain the appropriate volume and consistency of the blood. As pointed out in chapter 4, the kidneys control the amount of sodium and fluid retained in the body. In someone with normal blood pressure, the kidneys filter out excess sodium when there is too much in the blood, and when there is not enough, the kidneys reabsorb sodium from the urine and return it to the bloodstream. Individuals who have hypertension and a sensitivity to salt, however, retain more sodium than the body can use. When that happens, the blood pressure becomes elevated.

Although the actual physiological need for sodium may be as low as 220 milligrams a day, most Americans consume more than ten times that amount, from 2,500 milligrams (or 2.5 grams) and up each day. Sodium is most commonly found in table salt, which consists of 40 percent sodium and 60 percent chloride. The average adult American consumes anywhere from 5 to 20 grams of salt a day, which adds up to 2.5 to 8 grams of sodium. That is the equivalent of 1 to 4 teaspoons a day.

But table salt itself is only part of the sodium problem. Sodium occurs naturally in all foods. It exists in low quantities in fresh vegetables and fruit, seafood, and certain meats. Dairy products, you may be surprised to know, are fairly high in sodium. Foods that do not taste at all salty, such as bread and cookies, are also high in sodium, due in large part to the sodium content of baking soda and baking powder.

But for most people, the amount of sodium in these foods is not the culprit. Instead, it is the preponderance of processed food in the American diet that is implicated in our widespread hypertension problem. Canned vegetables and soups; frozen dinners; cured meats, including frankfurters, bacon, ham, and smoked fish; and the whole range of snack foods such as potato chips, pretzels, and crackers are all extraordinarily high in sodium. An ordinary frankfurter contains 500 milligrams of sodium; a hamburger in a fast-food restaurant could contain up to 1,000 milligrams of sodium.

Because there is no apparent risk to mild sodium restriction, whether or not you are salt sensitive, the most practical approach is to reduce the amount of sodium you consume to about 3 grams a day, which can usually be achieved by eliminating as many prepared foods as possible—especially snack foods and frozen meals—and all additions of salt to fresh food. (Fortunately, many manufacturers are now offering low-salt or salt-free frozen dinners, condiments, and other prepared foods. Purchase these alternatives whenever possible.) However, should you have severe hypertension that your physician feels is linked to salt sensitivity, he or she may recommend a salt-restricted diet. A moderate salt-restricted diet would involve reducing your sodium intake to 2,000 milligrams and a strict salt-restricted diet would mean lowering your intake to 1,000 milligrams each day.

Eating fresh vegetables and fruit, broiled chicken, a variety of complex carbohydrates such as pasta and rice, and using seasonings made without salt will go a long way in reducing your salt intake. Discuss with your doctor how salt may be affecting your high blood pressure. If you are one of the salt-sensitive hypertensives, there's a good chance that you could significantly reduce your blood pressure by restricting your sodium intake.

Reducing Fats and Cholesterol

A very important aspect of any eating plan is controlling the amount of fat and cholesterol consumed. Without limiting these substances, not only will you find weight loss to be nearly impossible but you will continue to damage your circulatory system, putting yourself at further risk for hypertension and stroke.

By reducing your dietary fat intake, you'll automatically reduce calories, which will lead to loss of excess weight. You'll also lower your risk for atherosclerosis— hypertension's deadly partner in the development of cardiovascular disease. Consuming too much dietary fat is directly related to the progression of atherosclerosis. Remember that many people who are not at all overweight consume too much cholesterol and fat, which then circulates through the bloodstream, damaging vessels along the way.

It should be noted at the start that when we talk about fat, we're usually discussing the larger category of body substances called lipids. Lipids include fats, fatty acids, and other compounds that are not soluble in water that circulate in our bloodstream and are part of our cells. Although not all lipids are fats, the two terms tend to be used interchangeably, which can be misleading. Cholesterol, for instance, is not a fat, but a fatlike lipid called a sterol.

Another misconception is that all stored fat is bad fat. In fact, stored body fat has important functions: it provides energy that can be released in times of need, it keeps the body warm, and it also provides a cushion for internal organs and bones. It is also a natural part of the human anatomy; more than 18 percent of the body weight of an average woman and 15 percent of the average man is made up of stored fat.

Fat has been proclaimed the great American food enemy. However, many people do not realize that a small amount of fat—about 1 tablespoon—must be consumed in the diet to provide essential fatty acids, which the body requires for a number of vital bodily functions. In addition, most people do not understand that not all fat is the same; in fact, there are a number of "good" fats that actually help us stay healthy. Basically, there are three different kinds of dietary fat, each with its own distinct properties:

- Saturated fats include animal products such as whole milk, some cheeses, butter, meat, cream, and hydrogenated vegetable shortenings; one way to recognize a saturated fat is that it is solid at room temperature. Saturated fats are the fats to avoid; they tend to raise the level of cholesterol in the blood by 5 to 10 percent. Cholesterol is discussed in detail later in this chapter.
- Unsaturated fats, also called polyunsaturated fats, include sunflower oil, corn oil, soybean oil, sesame oil, and other liquid fats of vegetable origin. These fats actually lower the amount of cholesterol in our bodies.
- Monounsaturated fats, like peanut oil and olive oil, also remain liquid at room temperature. These fats do not increase the amount of cholesterol or add to the amount of fat in the bloodstream; some studies indicate monounsaturated fats also help lower cholesterol levels.

Most fatty foods contain a combination of saturated and unsaturated fats, and all kinds of fats contain a large number of calories. For these two reasons, it's recommended that people who are eating for healthy heart, blood vessels, and blood pressure control limit the amount of fat to about 30 percent of a day's total calories (400 calories or less for those dieting to lose weight) and make sure only 10 percent of that amount consists of saturated fats.

What Is Cholesterol? Thanks in large part to efforts by the American Heart Association and other health organizations, Americans have become increasingly cholesterol conscious. In general, people are aware of the major fatty food risks—butter, eggs, cheese, and red meat. And yet, there is still a great deal of misconception about what cholesterol is and how it affects our circulatory system. Often the term lipid is used in describing fats. This is confusing. A lipid is any group of substances which cannot be dissolved in water. Fats, including cholesterol, are lipids. In the bloodstream the lipids are usually attached to other substances such as proteins and are called lipoproteins. It is the relationship between different kinds of lipoproteins that determines the amount of cholesterol circulating in the bloodstream.

These collections of fat and protein are characterized by their weight, or density. Low-density lipoproteins (LDLs) carry about two-thirds of circulating cholesterol to the cells; this is often the fat we speak of when referring to the plaque that builds up and causes atherosclerosis. High-density lipoproteins (HDLs) carry cholesterol away from the cells to the liver, where it is eliminated from the body. Very low density lipoproteins (VLDLs) carry saturated and unsaturated fats through the bloodstream. Therefore the high-density lipoproteins (HDLs) are acting to reduce the buildup of plaque and are nicknamed good cholesterol. The low-density lipoproteins are called bad cholesterol since they promote the formation of plaque.

Cholesterol is a fat found only in animal products like egg yolks, animal fats, cream, and cheese, to name just a few. Although, like fat, cholesterol is essential for a number of vital body processes, including nerve function and cell reproduction, there is no need for anyone to consume any cholesterol at all; the body manufactures all it needs. The average American, however, consumes anywhere from 600 to 1,500 milligrams of cholesterol each day.

We are born with about half of our cholesterol in the form of HDLs, but because the typical American diet is so high in saturated fats and cholesterol, we tend to replace HDLs with LDLs as we grow older. When you have more LDLs than HDLs, your body is transporting more cholesterol *into* the bloodstream, which increases your risk for atherosclerosis and heart disease, than out of the bloodstream. The role that VLDLs play in the development of atherosclerosis is not yet known, but a high level of VLDL indicates that there is too much fat in the bloodstream.

Of the blood lipids, most attention is paid to three

items when assessing their impact on cardiovascular and cerebrovascular health: total cholesterol, total fats, and the relationship between HDL and total cholesterol. The less cholesterol, fats, and LDL, the better. The more HDL that is circulating in the blood, the less cholesterol is available to form atherosclerosis.

The American Heart Association's Recommended Total Cholesterol Levels

Blood Cholesterol (in milligrams per deciliter)	Classification
200 or less	Desirable
200–239	Borderline high
240 and over	High

The amount of HDLs and LDLs that comprise your blood cholesterol greatly affects your risk of atherosclerosis and stroke. In general, the lower the LDLs and the higher the HDLs, the better. Ideally your LDL level should be below 130 milligrams per deciliter and your HDL level above 50 milligrams per deciliter. The lower your overall cholesterol levels are, the less risk you will run of having a complication of atherosclerosis such as stroke or heart attack.

The Risk Factors for High Cholesterol. Not surprisingly, the risk factors for high cholesterol are in great part mirror images of the risk factors of hypertension.

- *Heredity.* Genetics plays a certain, as yet not fully understood role in the development of high cholesterol. Some people can eat a high-fat, high-cholesterol diet and maintain normal blood cholesterol, while others have difficulty controlling cholesterol levels even when carefully monitoring their dietary intake.

  A clearer genetic factor is involved in rare conditions in which blood cholesterol and fat levels are extraordinarily high due to faulty metabolism. For people with these conditions, cholesterol-lowering drugs are usually prescribed in addition to diet, exercise, and other nondrug therapies.

- *Age.* Cholesterol levels tend to rise somewhat with age; those over fifty-five tend to have more circulating cholesterol than younger people, regardless of diet. However, recent studies have shown that children are not immune to high serum cholesterol levels; by some estimates, about 5 percent of American children from five to eighteen years have cholesterol levels over 200.

  Atherosclerosis is known for being a "slow" disease; it often takes years for the damage to blood vessels to cause overt symptoms. That's why the American Heart Association recently recommended that children in families with a history of cardiovascular disease be examined by their doctors and put on a corrective diet if their blood lipid levels are excessive.

- *Obesity.* Overweight people tend to have both high levels of total cholesterol and low levels of HDL, the protective lipoproteins that remove fat and cholesterol from the body. Usually, sensible dieting corrects both weight and blood lipid levels.
- *Gender.* Men generally have higher HDL and total cholesterol levels than do women, although women nearly catch up after menopause.

Reducing the amount of cholesterol and fat in your diet, whether or not you have any predisposing risk factors of hypertension, is one of the best ways to reduce your risk of atherosclerosis, which is, as we've discussed, accelerated and exacerbated by hypertension. Cholesterol is found in a wide variety of foods, and it is quite easy to consume far too much of it if you're not careful. One egg yolk, for instance, contains 250 to 275 milligrams of cholesterol; two eggs for breakfast means that you're already over your limit for the day. In addition to the well-publicized culprits like fried foods, eggs, red meat, cheese, and butter, other, not so obvious foods—like shrimp—are also high in cholesterol.

Other Dietary Considerations

Potassium. A chemical essential for muscle contraction and other body functions, potassium also plays a role in helping the kidneys eliminate sodium from the body. In fact, many causes of secondary hypertension, such as primary aldosteronism (in which the body produces too much of the hormone aldosterone) and Cushing's disease (in which the body produces too much of the hormone hydrocortisone), involve *hypokalemia,* or low levels of potassium.

Is it possible to prevent essential hypertension or to control moderate cases simply by consuming more potassium? Probably not. But, interestingly enough, potassium is most often found in food low in sodium, so that when you reduce your intake of sodium, you often automatically increase your intake of potassium. The use of potassium supplements is highly controversial, because too much potassium (hyperkalemia) can cause serious illness. Discuss whether or not you need extra potassium with your physician before taking supplements.

Calcium. Supplemental calcium in the diet has been found to lower blood pressure in some patients. This added calcium may be in pills, food additives, or in foods naturally high in calcium. In addition to milk products, other foods such as figs and green leafy vegetables are a good source of calcium (and high in fiber as well).

Alcohol. Alcohol is under investigation for its role in hypertension. Heavy drinking causes hypertension in many individuals. If an individual with normal blood pressure drinks more than 2 ounces of alcohol a day on a regular basis, his or her blood pressure rises. However, a limit of 2 ounces of alcohol or less should have no effect on blood pressure; some studies have shown that moderate drinking seems to provide some protection against heart attacks and strokes.

Caffeine. Caffeine is another dietary hazard; it is a stimulant that causes a temporary rise in blood pressure and heart action. Is a moderate amount of caffeine considered a risk factor for hypertension stroke? No. While drinking two or three cups of coffee, for instance, may cause an elevation in arterial pressure for an hour or two, it usually drops back to normal after that. However, if you are hypertensive, discuss this with your doctor. In some patients the temporary rise in blood pressure may be exaggerated.

Diet for Life

In general, the old adage "everything in moderation" remains true in terms of diet to prevent and control hypertension. Learning about proper nutrition and following a sound eating plan will go a long way in reducing our risk for cardiovascular disease. To get you started, take another look at the American Heart Association's dietary guidelines, listed on page 81. If you follow these recommendations, you should slowly but surely lose weight and improve your cardiovascular health.

For the average person, however, trying to figure out what percentage of daily calories is being derived from proteins, carbohydrates, or fats is often troublesome and complicated. A simpler method is to go back to the old-fashioned "four basic food groups" idea, keeping in mind that to achieve safe weight loss, about 1,200 to 1,800 calories per day should be consumed.

This will result in about a 1 to 2 pound drop per week. Consult your doctor about the proper amount of calorie consumption, based on your current weight and how many pounds you would like to lose.

The following daily portions of fruits, vegetables, breads, protein, dairy products, and fat will start you on your way to a healthier body.

- Aim for 4 to 6 ounces of protein; this includes egg whites as desired, but only two to three whole eggs per week (chicken, turkey, fish, lean beef, veal, pork, lamb, lentils, dried peas, sprouts, grains, and nuts are protein foods).
- Have three servings of ½ cup or more of fresh vegetables.
- Eat three servings of medium-size fruit.
- Include four servings of bread/starches, each serving limited to no more than 80 calories (bread, English muffins, pasta, cereal, potatoes, rice, rice cakes, and popcorn are good choices).
- Consume two 8-ounce servings of low-fat milk, yogurt, or cottage cheese; this includes hard cheeses, but no more than four 1-ounce servings per week.
- Eat no more than 2 tablespoons of fat.

Using this plan, the often tedious struggle of counting calories and dieting is replaced by the more natural approach of portion control and food variety.

Before undertaking any eating plan, however, you should consult with your physician. That is especially true for anyone with diabetes or other disorders that are affected by diet.

Exercise and Hypertension

At the beginning of this century more than half of all Americans worked in jobs such as agriculture, construction, and so forth—that met their daily exercise needs. When our great-grandparents and grandparents were growing up, no one joined a health club or took up jogging and there were no more fat people then than there are now. Today, fewer than 2 percent of the U.S. population has jobs that involve any kind of cardiovascular effort. The problems related to this sedentary lifestyle continue to grow. According to a study by the President's Council on Fitness conducted in the mid-1980s, about 55 percent of Americans take part in some form of physical exercise, but less than one-third of us do enough exercise to derive any health benefits from it.

The role of exercise in the prevention and treatment of cardiovascular disease is a subject of increasing interest to both the general public and the medical profession. At one time, most hypertensive and even potentially hypertensive patients were told not to exert themselves for fear of provoking a stroke or heart attack. More and more, however, exercise conditioning is not only strongly recommended as a preventive measure, but is frequently used a rehabilitative method in working with stroke and heart attack patients.

How does exercise improve cardiovascular health? One link is between exercise and weight reduction—the more you exercise, the more calories you burn, helping you to lose extra pounds. In addition, a number of studies have found that regular, vigorous exercise increases levels of HDL. The beneficial effect of higher HDL is lower total blood cholesterol and an increase in the ratio of HDLs to total cholesterol. As pointed out previously, this reduces the risk for atherosclerosis. Diabetics and hypertensive patients who regularly exercise are often able to reduce their medication dramatically.

Your heart also benefits from a good workout: Because your muscles need more oxygen when they are at work, the heart must pump harder to get extra oxygen-rich blood to them. Normally, the heart pumps about 6 quarts of blood a minute in an average adult man, but when the body is exercising, blood volume to and from the heart rises to about 25 quarts per minute. This extra work strengthens the heart muscle; the stronger it is, the less hard it has to work to meet the body's need for oxygen. Exercise also helps improve the health of the entire circulatory system.

The First Steps to Exercise

Even if your blood pressure level is normal, before you start exercising you must first consult with your physician.

He or she may recommend a stress test to see how your heart and blood vessels are functioning. A stress test involves nothing more than having your heart rate measured by *electrocardiography* (EKG) and your blood pressure monitored by a technician while you jog on a treadmill or ride a stationary bicycle. One of the most important benefits of the stress test is that it helps diagnose heart and vessel disease through changes in the EKG tracings. It will also help determine the amount of exercise your heart and muscles can handle without any adverse effects. If you should, at any time, during the stress test or during any other period of physical activity, experience any of the following symptoms, *stop exercising immediately:*

- Chest discomfort, including pain, tightness, heaviness, or breathlessness.
- Any discomfort or numbness in the jaw, neck, or arm.
- Dizziness.
- Headache.
- Nausea.

Both the length of time you are able to exercise during the stress test and the intensity of activity you are able to endure without becoming tired will help your doctor determine a safe exercise routine for you.

In order for exercise to have a healthy effect on the cardiovascular system, it must be of a sufficient intensity and frequency. Thus the next step is to determine your target heart rate, or the rate at which your heart must work to provide health benefits to the cardiovascular system. Your target heart rate is between 70 and 85 percent of your maximum heart rate; your maximum heart rate is calculated by subtracting your age from 220 (see Table 4). For the average thirty-year-old, the maximum heart rate would be $220 - 30 = 190$. This individual's target heart rate range is from 133 to 162 beats per minute, which is 70 to 85 percent of the maximum heart rate. You can determine whether or not you are within your target zone by taking your pulse immediately after exercise.

The easiest way to take your pulse is to place two fingers (not your thumb; it is also a pulse point and can disturb the accuracy of your reading) on one of your *carotid arteries,* which are located to the left and

Table 4.
Finding Your Target Heart Rate

Age	Target Zone*	Maximum Heart Rate[a]
20	140–170	200
25	137–166	195
30	133–162	190
35	130–157	185
40	126–153	180
45	123–149	175
50	119–145	170
55	116–140	165
60	112–136	160
65	109–132	155
70	105–128	150

*Measured in beats per minute.
Remember: The easiest way to check your pulse rate is to count the beats for fifteen seconds then multiply by four. This will give you beats per minute.

right of your throat in the neck. Count the beats for fifteen seconds, then multiply that number by four. If your pulse rate is below the target range, you should increase either the intensity or the length of your workout. If your pulse is above your target rate, slow down.

Choosing an Exercise Program
What kind of exercise should you do? In general, if you're at risk for hypertension, you should concentrate on aerobic exercise. Aerobic exercise consists of moving the large muscle groups freely, generating heat in the

body, and thus burning up oxygen. Swimming, jogging, cycling, singles tennis, skiing, rowing, dancing—any of these activities, done regularly, will boost your heart rate.

Please note that isometric exercise, also known as weight training, is *not* recommended for someone with very high blood pressure. The tensing of the muscles in the arms and legs causes a restriction of the blood vessels, a reduction in the flow of blood, and can lead to problems. However, if your blood pressure is normal or even borderline, weight training may be perfectly appropriate for you. Ask your physician for advice.

How often should you exercise? The optimal frequency for those beginning an exercise program is three to four times a week; if you need to lose weight, four to five times a week is recommended. Each period of exercise should last from thirty to forty-five minutes each, but beginners should start out exercising for just five to ten minutes, slowly increasing the amount of time until the target rate is reached. Optimally, you should exercise at your target rate from fifteen to twenty-five minutes, with a ten-minute warm-up and ten-minute cool-down period. If you are a beginner, please consult your physician for guidelines.

How long should your exercise program last? Forever. Regular exercise must become a part of your daily life if lasting health benefits are to be derived. Therefore, perhaps the most important element in the design of your exercise program is choosing activities you will enjoy over the long haul. Very often, people start exercising with great enthusiasm, but after just a few weeks revert to their former sedentary ways. Boredom, inconvenience, and lack of motivation are commonly listed reasons given by former exercisers for quitting.

To alleviate boredom, you may want to alternate activities: take a dance class one session, bicycle for forty-five minutes the next, play a game of tennis the next. As long as you reach and sustain your target heart rate for thirty minutes or more, it doesn't matter what form of exercise you choose.

Another hint to help you stick to an exercise program is to eliminate as many excuses as possible for not exercising. If you join a health club that is only open during hours you are at work, for instance, then obviously you are setting yourself up to fail. Scheduling times to exercise—and treating your exercise times as if they were business appointments—is often the only way to incorporate exercise into your lifestyle.

For most of us, there comes a time when our motivation sags and we lose interest in exercising on a regular basis. When this happens—preferably *before* this happens—enlist a friend or loved one to join you in your quest for cardiovascular health. Often, a little competition and companionship goes a long way. Support from your spouse, family, and friends is critical. It is easier to keep the program going if a family member or friend is enrolled with you.

Getting enough exercise doesn't have to be very complicated. The American Medical Association has pointed out that a walk of just 1 mile a day at a moderate pace for thirty-six days is a simple and pleasant way to lose 1 pound of fat and give your heart a decent workout. After a year, you will have lost 10 pounds and incorporated exercise into your life very simply.

Keep in mind that exercise has psychological as well as physiological benefits. People who exercise find they not only feel better physically but also have a renewed sense of emotional well-being. Part of the reason is that certain body chemicals called endorphins, known to dull pain and produce a mild euphoria, are released during vigorous exercise. Smokers who exercise find it easier to quit, therapists frequently prescribe exercise to their depressed patients, and dieters who also exercise claim to feel less hungry than they did when they were sedentary. Another most important benefit of regular aerobic workouts is that they seem to reduce stress—an especially important consideration for hypertensive patients.

Stress and Hypertension

There is little doubt that our psychological state has an effect on our physical body. How much do our emotions affect our health? A comprehensive answer to that question is not yet available. It is known that for most people hypertension is *not* caused solely by tension or stress. Many people who eventually develop high blood pressure are calm, easygoing, and enjoy a relatively tension-free lifestyle.

The problem in correlating stress and health is two-

fold. First, except for extreme situations, like the death
of a loved one or divorce, a clear definition of stress
itself is not available. One man's day at the beach could
be sheer torture for someone whose idea of fun is a day
making business deals at the office. Also, many of us
define stress far too narrowly: stress is physical as well
as emotional—your body experiences stress every time
you shovel snow or carry a sack of groceries up a flight
of stairs. When you make love, for instance, your body
is also under stress; hormones are being stimulated,
heart rate and blood pressure are increased, and muscles
are tensed. Stress can be positive as well as negative.
The emotions attached to the birth of a child may create
as much stress on you as the death of a spouse, but the
nature of the stress and the reaction to it is quite
different.

Second, not everyone responds to stress in the same
way; some people become outwardly aggravated over
the slightest mishap while others never blink an eye
even when disaster occurs. But it could be that the outwardly calm person is seething inside, driving up his or
her blood pressure to even higher levels than the person
who expresses anger and frustration in a more open
way. Many of these controlled people are not aware of
the enormous tension they experience by this sublima-
tion of their emotions.

As you can see, defining stress and its relationship to
hypertension that leads to stroke is not an easy task. A
great deal of research, however, has indicated that there
may indeed be a very important connection. One of the
most controversial theories, first developed by Dr.

Meyer Friedman and Dr. Ray Rosenman, concerning stress and disease divided Americans into Type A (demanding and ambitious) and Type B (calm and easygoing) personalities. In a study conducted at Duke University in North Carolina, more than 3,000 men—approximately 1,500 Type A's and 1,500 Type B's—were followed to see the effect their personalities had on their health.

After eight years, it was found that Type A men had significantly more atherosclerosis than Type B men. Data on how this development might affect their potential specifically for hypertension were not collected. However, it was calculated that the increase in atherosclerosis put the Type A men at twice the risk for having a heart attack than the Type B men. Subsequent studies have focused on the fact that there are Type A women who suffer the same health-related problems as Type A males.

While these studies and many others have indicated that stress is related to cardiovascular health, the extent and the manner of its effect is still largely unknown. How could personality affect blood pressure levels? The connection between the two seems to be the ways in which certain people produce the fight or flight stress hormones, norepinephrine and epinephrine, as well as cortisol and testosterone. Rises in the levels of stress-related hormones vary from person to person: in some people, the hormonal responses are brief, while in others, the altered levels may persist longer.

These hormones, as we discussed in chapter 2, are

released by the adrenal medulla when danger or stress is sensed by the brain. The job of epinephrine and nor-epinephrine is to stimulate heart and blood vessel action, in effect preparing the body for a physical fight against the perceived stress. Animal experiments with the hormone cortisol, for instance, have shown that an increase in cortisol raises the level of cholesterol and other lipids in the blood. This, of course, paves the way for atherosclerosis.

The Fine Art of Relaxing

For many individuals, rest and relaxation do not come easily. In fact, for many people, *trying* to relax can be a stressful activity in itself. If you relate relaxation with laziness, for instance, it is unlikely that you will be able to help control your blood pressure by taking a nap every afternoon.

During the past decade, considerable interest has been directed toward the question of whether the effects of stress on blood pressure could be modified. *Biofeedback* is one method that has received a good deal of attention. It was developed after studies showed that animals could control their autonomic functions, like blood pressure, by being given a reward or a punishment. Physicians adapted those findings to design ways for humans to control unconscious functions through conscious thought.

There are many biofeedback methods. One involves monitoring patients with a machine equipped with lights similar to traffic lights. A special blood pressure cuff that has a microphone that will project the sound of any changes in blood pressure is attached to the patient's arm. As blood pressure rises, the lights on the machine as well as the sounds being emitted by the microphone let the patient monitor his or her own blood pressure. If it goes too high, for instance, the machine's lights may blink red, if pressure is normal, the light will turn yellow, if it's too low, it may blink green. The patient can learn to control the blood pressure by consciously calming down if the pressure is too high, or by thinking about stressful situations if the pressure is too low. The goal is for the patient to continue this method of blood pressure control without the need for the monitoring machine.

Not all solutions to the stress problem are so elaborate. For some, daily exercise will eliminate stress, while for others meditation is the answer. The relaxation response, developed by Boston physician Dr. Herbert Benson in the 1970s, relies on the tradition of transcendental meditation to evoke a calm, relaxed attitude in patients who are under stress.

Relaxation Exercise

There are many relaxation exercises that will help relieve tension; the following is used quite often by physicians and therapists to treat stress.

1. Sit or lie down in a comfortable position in a quiet, dimly lit room.
2. Close your eyes and breathe deeply and regularly,

concentrating only on the sound of your breathing. Try to shut out all other thoughts.

3. Now, as you take your next deep breath, allow the muscles in your feet and ankles to relax and actually picture in your mind that part of your body sinking into the chair, floor, or bed. Sometimes it is helpful to first tense the muscles in the feet and then release them; this helps you to remember the feeling of relaxing.

4. Continue the process, always breathing deeply and regularly, relaxing each part of your body from your calves to your knees, thighs, hips, stomach, chest, shoulders, arms, hands, neck, and face.

Take as much time as possible, but no less than fifteen minutes. By the end of the exercise, you should feel relaxed and calm.

Although these methods are receiving a great deal of well-deserved attention, you should be aware that for the average hypertensive patient they have not been proven to significantly decrease arterial pressure levels on a permanent basis.

Cigarette Smoking

Cigarette smoking is the most important proven cause of premature death in the United States, accounting for approximately 250,000 of the 2 million overall deaths each year. About 35 percent of all smokers die prematurely of a smoking-related disease. Smokers are three times more likely to die of cancer than nonsmokers. The Framingham Heart Study found that men who smoke are ten times as likely to experience sudden death from cardiac arrest as nonsmokers. Among women smokers, the mortality rate is five times greater for sudden death.

The combination of cigarette smoking and hypertension increases the risk of stroke and heart attack considerably. If you know you have a genetic predisposition to hypertension and you smoke cigarettes, you have greatly increased your risk for having a fatal cardiovascular disease.

How Cigarette Smoke Kills

There are some 4,000 substances identified in cigarette smoke—some highly toxic and carcinogenic (cancer causing). One of the most deadly substances ingested by man, nicotine, is cigarette smoke's main component. What does nicotine do to the body? When you puff a cigarette, nicotine immediately enters the bloodstream and reaches the brain within six seconds, where more than 15 percent of it is absorbed. Nicotine is a stimulant; when it reaches the brain, it signals the adrenal glands to release norepinephrine and epinephrine (adrenaline), which increase both the systolic and diastolic pressure. Nicotine is absorbed in the mouth as well as the lungs. Therefore, even if you don't inhale, large amounts of nicotine still enter the bloodstream. Your heart beats faster, it pumps more blood, and your arteries work harder to push the blood through your body. This elevates the blood pressure and contributes to blood vessel atherosclerosis.

In addition to directly causing an increase in heart and vessel activity, cigarette smoking also contributes to the advance of atherosclerosis, hypertension's deadly partner. First, nicotine is known to raise the amount of fats and cholesterol circulating in the bloodstream by releasing some of the stored body fat. This increase in circulating fats also contributes to the process that forms plaque on artery walls. Cigarette smoking has been shown to raise the level of low-density lipoproteins (the bad cholesterol) by as much as 10 percent. Second, another ingredient of cigarette smoke, carbon dioxide, helps the process along by directly damaging the cells that form the inner linings of arterial walls. This makes the vessel lining more susceptible to plaque buildup.

To compound the situation further, the carbon dioxide, a toxic gas, is carried through the bloodstream by the same blood component, hemoglobin, that transports oxygen. The more carbon dioxide in the bloodstream, therefore, the less oxygen is being carried to the vital organs. While nicotine stimulates heart and vessel activity, carbon monoxide prevents oxygen from helping the body do this extra work.

Cigarette smoking also causes chemical changes in the blood itself, causing it to become more viscous, or sticky, which results in the formation of large blood clots, a process called thrombosis. These clots can cause both strokes and heart attacks.

Cigarette smoking may also increase the risk of developing renovascular hypertension, a form of secondary hypertension involving the kidneys. Tobacco smoke also contains cadmium, a substance known to contribute directly to the development of high blood pressure. When cadmium is inhaled through smoking, it tends to be retained in the kidneys, further increasing hypertension levels.

Why Do We Smoke?

Since the dangers of smoking were made public by the surgeon general in 1964, almost 50 million people have stopped smoking for good. Some people cite the fact that so many people no longer smoke as a way to account for at least part of the decrease in the number of cardiovascular deaths in the last two decades.

Unfortunately, for every smoker who stops, someone else picks up this dangerous habit. Teenage girls seem to be the most susceptible to the lure of cigarette smoking; in fact, in the last decade, lung cancer has surpassed breast cancer as the leading cause of cancer death in women. This statistic is directly related to the changing smoking habits of women.

The American Heart Association, the surgeon general of the United States, the American Cancer Society, and countless other professional organizations and physicians all concur:

If you smoke now, you must quit in order to live a full and healthy life.

Ample evidence proves that the risk of developing cardiovascular disease is reduced by 20 to 50 percent within five years of stopping smoking.

Is knowing the dangers of smoking often not enough to make someone stop smoking? There is one important reason: The smoker is addicted to the powerful drug nicotine. The longer a person has smoked and the more he or she has smoked, the stronger the addiction. In a 1988 report, the surgeon general concluded that nicotine is not only addictive but is addictive in the same way as are other narcotics, like heroin and cocaine. People who smoke become increasingly tolerant to the effects of nicotine, needing more cigarettes to satisfy their craving for the drug. If they quit smoking, they experience classic drug withdrawal symptoms—nausea, fatigue, anxiety, insomnia, and irritability.

It is a fact that up to 70 percent of all those who quit will at one time or another relapse and begin smoking again. But that is not to say that quitting is impossible. Just think of the nearly 50 million people who have stopped—and lived healthier lives because of it.

A good first step in deciding when and how to quit is to figure out *exactly why* you smoke. The American Cancer Society and the U.S. Public Health Service Clearing House for Smoking has defined six types of smokers and their behaviors.

- *Addicts*. Addictive smokers are both physically and psychologically dependent on cigarettes. They usually start craving their next cigarette as soon as they have put one out. Many addicts find that chewing nicotine-laced gum during the withdrawal process is helpful. See your physician if you find the phys-

ical part of your addiction to cigarettes overwhelming.

- *Handlers.* For the handling smoker, it is not so
much the inhaling of the cigarette as it is having
something to do with his or her hands. Handlers
should keep swizzle sticks, paper clips, or other
hand toys within reach whenever the urge to smoke
overtakes them.

- *Habit smokers.* Some smokers will light up cigarette
after cigarette without even realizing that they are
smoking. If they ever had experienced any real pleas-
ure from smoking, these smokers have long ceased
to feel it. For them, smoking is merely a habit they
cannot control. Replacing old habits with new ones
is by no means easy, but many ex-smokers have reported that taking up a sport or a hobby made the
transition to nonsmoking much easier.

- *Crutch smokers.* Smoking to relieve tension is one of
the most common reasons given for cigarette addiction. Smokers who use cigarettes as a crutch during
times of stress will light up at the first sign of trouble.
Exercise is a sure-fire way to reduce stress; many ex-
smokers who smoked out of nervousness find that a
brisk walk or run releases some of their pent-up frustration. Crutch smokers often find a release in the
same hand toys as do handlers; fidgeting with a paper clip reduces a surprising amount of tension.

- *Stimulation seekers.* Looking for a lift that they believe comes only with a cigarette, these smokers will
claim that smoking helps them think more clearly

and act more decisively. For the stimulation seeker, too, exercise is a good replacement for cigarettes. Running can especially provide the same kind of physical high ex-smokers used to get from nicotine.

• *Relaxation seekers.* "Nothing makes me feel better than smoking a cigarette" is the oft-heard refrain from those smokers who use cigarettes to enhance other pleasurable experiences like eating, drinking, and sex. In many ways, this is the most difficult hurdle to get over, because you would not want to avoid your favorite activities in order to stop smoking. It may be best to change the pattern of those activities to make smoking difficult. Have drinks in the no-smoking section of a restaurant instead of a bar; take a long walk after dinner instead of smoking; have sex in the morning, when there is not as much time to relax—or crave a cigarette—afterward.

No matter why you smoke, quitting is probably not going to be easy for you. As you struggle to overcome your addiction, keep in mind that you will be improving your chances of avoiding the stroke that you may be predisposed to having through your family history.

Kicking the Habit

Studies have shown that 95 percent of all people who quit smoking do it on their own, going cold turkey. Other methods, such as antismoking pills or nicotine gum prescribed by a physician, techniques like Smoke-Enders, or hypnosis have also proven to be quite effective. Both the American Heart Association (see box on page 121) and the American Cancer Society have drawn up plans to help those who want to quit find the will-power and the strength to do so.

For most people, however, stopping smoking is one of the most difficult tasks they've ever attempted. Many people actually feel physically ill for a week or two after they stop. Why? Because they are actually experiencing withdrawal from the powerful drug nicotine. You may feel nervous and irritable. You may have headaches, muscle cramping, and be unable to sleep. Physicians recommend drinking extra amounts of water and other fluids—up to ten glasses a day—to help flush the nicotine out of the kidneys. Try to avoid caffeinated coffees and teas; they will only make you even more nervous.

Like exercise or dieting, becoming a nonsmoker takes time and energy. The first three months—before not smoking becomes as much a part of your life as smoking had been—are often the toughest. It is during this time that most ex-smokers start smoking again, especially if other stresses in life, like a divorce or difficulties at work, intrude.

Indeed, failure rates among smokers are quite high. If you are a smoker, no doubt you have tried many times to stop. Here are some hints that might make your struggle to stop smoking a little easier to bear.

- Make a list of all the places you go where you do not smoke. Spend as much time as possible in those places. These days it is getting easier and easier to

The American Heart Association's Four-Step Quit Smoking Program

Even before you quit altogether, there are things you can do to prepare yourself.

1. *List all the positive reasons why you want to quit smoking and read the list daily.* Wrap your cigarette pack with paper and rubber bands. Each time you smoke, unwrap the pack to remove a cigarette, write down the time of day, what you are doing, how you feel, and how important that cigarette is to you on a scale from one to five. Then rewrap the pack before you smoke the cigarette. Keep reading your list of reasons and add to it if possible.

2. *Don't carry matches and keep your cigarettes some distance away from you.* Try keeping them in a drawer or on the top shelf of a closet. Each day try to smoke fewer cigarettes; take a look at your schedule of cigarettes and eliminate either the ones most important to you or least important, depending on which is most effective.

3. *Continue with step 2.* Don't buy a new pack until you finish the one you're smoking. And never buy a carton. Change brands twice during the week, each time choosing a brand lower in nicotine and tar, a mixture of several substances that condense into a sticky substance in the lungs. Tar is a carcinogen, a cancer-causing

agent. Try to stop smoking for twenty-four to
forty-eight hours during this period.

4. *Quit smoking entirely.* Increase your physical
   activity. Avoid situations you most closely associate with cigarettes. Do deep breathing exercises whenever you get the urge to smoke.
   Find a substitute for cigarettes: sugarless gum,
   hard candy, or toothpicks, for example.

find such places: museums, department stores, con-
cert halls, and movie theaters are just a few of the
pleasant places to spend time where you cannot do
the one thing you are probably yearning to do:
smoke. On the other hand, taking the time to spend
a lovely afternoon looking at fine works of art, trying on beautiful clothes, or seeing a hit movie takes
the bite out of not lighting up. Today, almost all
restaurants have nonsmoking sections; treat yourself to an elegant lunch or dinner—just make sure
you sit where smoking a cigarette is impossible.
Spend time with nonsmoking friends.

- Instead of smoking after meals, get up from the table and brush your teeth or go for a walk. Just
  getting up from the table will help; if you brush
  your teeth, you'll be less likely to smoke; walking
  will take your mind off your craving for nicotine.
- Take public transportation. Does starting the car
  mean lighting up a cigarette? For many people,
  smoking while driving is an ingrained habit. If
  that's true for you, start to take public transporta-

tion as often as possible. Buses and subways are off-limits to smoking so you'll be disassociating yourself from another situation in which you might be tempted to smoke.

• Create a clean, smoke-free environment at home. You will notice immediately how fresh your clothes and furniture smell, how clean your teeth and breath are, how much more appealing a house without ashes and ashtrays can be.

Does Quitting Smoking Mean Gaining Weight?

For those patients who are overweight and trying to prevent high blood pressure or are trying to lower their blood pressure, this is indeed a most important question. It is true that many people turn to food as a substitute for cigarettes and gain a few pounds. But that should not stop you from quitting for a number of reasons.

First of all, studies have shown that the average weight gain when a person stops smoking is only 5 to 10 pounds, and some of this weight gain may be temporary, caused by increased fluid retention during the withdrawal period. Second, it is far less dangerous to your health to put on a few extra pounds than to continue to smoke. In fact, according to the American Heart Association, it would take the addition of about 75 to 100 pounds to negate the health benefits that a normal smoker gains by quitting.

It is true, however, that your metabolism may change somewhat when you quit smoking; you may find yourself not able to eat quite as much as you could while

smoking without gaining some weight. The oral grati-
fication aspect of smoking—simply enjoying having
something in your mouth—may cause you to turn to
food when you no longer can reach for a cigarette.

A more positive factor in an ex-smoker's potential
weight gain is the brand-new sense of taste that goes
along with quitting smoking. Ex-smokers often remark
on how good food tastes when the nicotine and other
chemicals no longer tinge the taste buds. This can work
to your advantage, however, when you rediscover how
delicious fresh fruits and vegetables—and other low-
calorie/low-fat foods—really taste. In addition to following some of the dietary tips you read about earlier
in this chapter, you might consider keeping healthy
snacks around the house (unsalted, unbuttered popcorn, sugarless candy and gum, and fresh vegetables
and fruit).

Perhaps most important of all, consult your doctor
and start an exercise program. Not only will a brisk
walk or bicycle ride after every meal do wonders for
your cardiovascular health in general but it will take
your mind off the after-dinner smoke that had become
a deadly habit. Take a look at the section on exercise
(page 101) to find other reasons to exchange the bad
habit of cigarette smoking for the good one of exercise.

A Lifelong Commitment

As discussed at the end of chapter 1, the prevention of
hypertension requires a lifelong commitment. Reducing

your risk for hypertension involves incorporating healthier eating, exercise, and stress-reduction habits into your *daily* routine. For some, making these changes is much harder than for others; for those people, medical treatment involving drugs and, in some rare instances, surgery is recommended.

Indeed, although some of the recent dramatic decline in the incidence of hypertension, stroke, and heart attack can be linked to our new attention to a healthier lifestyle, much of the success belongs to the advances made in drug and surgical treatment for both cardiovascular disease in general and stroke in particular. In the next chapter, you'll learn about both the benefits and the side effects of medical antihypertensive therapy.

Questions and Answers

Q: Will having a glass of wine or a Scotch every evening after work relax me enough to lower my blood pressure?

A. While having 1 or 2 ounces of alcohol a day should not harm you under most circumstances, it would be a mistake to think that the feelings of relaxation that accompany taking a drink will do anything to permanently lower blood pressure. In fact, heavy drinking raises the blood pressure, and the extra calories involved can exacerbate obesity, increasing another risk factor for stroke.

Q: I want to lose weight, both because I feel too heavy and because I've been diagnosed with borderline hypertension. I've been eating low-calorie frozen dinners on many evenings when I work late. Am I doing the right thing?

A: By trying to lose weight, absolutely. By eating frozen dinners? Probably not. While the low calories may help you to lose weight, you may be adding another considerable risk factor to your hypertension: high sodium intake. Some frozen dinners can contain as many as 2,000 milligrams of sodium and up, which means you'll exceed your total daily amount of sodium in just one meal. Many frozen food producers, aware of the public's increasing concern over sodium levels, now sell low-sodium, low-calorie dinners.

Make sure you read the labels of all foods carefully so you don't sabotage your good efforts to lower your risk for stroke.

Q: My wife frequently works late and is always on a deadline. But her blood pressure is normal and she says she feels as healthy as an ox. Should I worry about her developing hypertension?

A: The relationship between stress and hypertension is one of the least understood in this very complicated syndrome. Some studies have shown that it is not the *amount* of stress you are under that determines your risk for disease, but how much *control* you feel over what's causing the stress. White-collar executives, for instance, who have high-pressure jobs but who are in positions of authority, develop hypertension at lower rates than blue-collar workers, who feel a lack of control over their situations. Stress is a very individual phenomenon; your wife may very well thrive, healthy and safe, under circumstances many of us would find intolerable.

6

Controlling Hypertension
with Drugs

So far in this book, we've concentrated on factors that influence the development of hypertension and how to eliminate or modify them. If you've worked hard enough on reducing your risk factors and have managed to maintain your blood pressure within the normal range, you may be able to skip this chapter altogether.

Hundreds of thousands of Americans are diagnosed with high blood pressure every year. Some of them may have even struggled to make the lifestyle changes described in chapter 5 work for them. Despite their best efforts, however, their blood pressure has risen above the normal zone into the danger zone of hypertension. Perhaps they just could not lose that 20 pounds or exercise on a regular basis. Or perhaps their uncontrollable risk factors, such as increasing age and a genetic predisposition, were overwhelming.

If you have been diagnosed with hypertension, don't

despair. You are not doomed to suffer serious cardio-vascular disease; there are many treatment options open to someone with high blood pressure. If your blood pressure reading is between 140/90 and 159/94 milli-meters of mercury, for instance, you may be able to manage your condition with the same diet and exercise plans outlined in chapter 5.

If your blood pressure reading is 160/95 or above, however, you and your doctor may decide that drug therapy is necessary. As stated in chapter 1, research on antihypertensive drugs during the last two or three de-cades has produced some very effective medications that lower blood pressure safely. Some 30 million people take blood pressure medication today.

What factors determine when drug therapy is neces-sary in a particular case of hypertension? The decision depends on how many other risk factors for cardiovas-cular disease, particularly heart attack and stroke, are present in the hypertensive patient and the intensity of the pressure readings. Symptoms directly related to se-vere hypertension such as dizziness, chest pains, or se-vere headache mandate immediate drug therapy.

It probably will not surprise you that the risk factors of these diseases mirror those of hypertension: namely, high cholesterol, obesity, sedentary lifestyle, smoking, diabetes, and a family history of cardiovascular disease. If one or more of these risk factors are present *and* you also have high blood pressure, your doctor is far more likely to prescribe antihypertensive drugs to you than if you were in better shape. (All the more reason to follow the antihypertensive game plan discussed in chapter 5!)

A logical question to ask is, "If drugs are available to treat hypertension, then why bother trying to prevent or lower blood pressure by changing my lifestyle?" Although antihypertensive medications are quite effective, they are not without their disadvantages. Because the blood pressure control is a lifelong proposition, most patients who rely on medication must take one or more pills each day, every day, for the rest of their lives. As hard as it is to learn new lifestyle habits, such as lowering salt and fat intake and exercising regularly, so it is to learn to take a drug, or even a combination of drugs, every day. This is especially true for hypertension patients, who often experience no symptoms of their disease. In addition, antihypertensive drugs cost money. Each pill may not be terribly costly, but two or three pills each day for 365 days a year can run up a bill.

The matter is further complicated by the fact that many of these drugs have unpleasant side effects that range from lethargy and weakness to impotence and depression. Indeed, it is ironic that hypertension itself usually produces no symptoms at all but the drugs used to control it often make the patient feel ill; this is the main reason so many people fail to control their high blood pressure successfully with drugs. In fact, according to surveys conducted by the National Health and Nutrition Examination, only about three out of five hypertensives on drug therapy have their blood pressure under control.

Why? First, as discussed above, it is difficult for some people to get used to taking pills every day. And second, the side effects, when they occur, can be discouraging and frustrating. But you must keep in mind that although you may have never *felt* ill in the past your high blood pressure may have been causing severe damage to your cardiovascular system—damage that might end up costing you brain or heart function or your life.

If you've been diagnosed with high blood pressure in the moderate range, *must* you take medication? Not necessarily. Many patients in the moderate range can get by without any drugs—if they work hard enough to control their weight and diet. Whether drug therapy, lifestyle modifications, or a combination of the two will work best for you is a decision that you and your physician should reach together.

Like any other drugs, those that treat hypertension will affect your body in a number of different ways, and if you or someone you are close to has been diagnosed with hypertension, you'll want to learn as much as you can about both the benefits and drawbacks of drug therapy.

When beginning an antihypertensive drug therapy, all patients should see their physicians frequently, sometimes every week or two. You should tell your doctor *every* side effect you have; don't worry how major or minor it seems. Any number of alternate therapies may be available to you if one drug or drug combination makes you feel uncomfortable. Once the decision is made to begin drug therapy, *do not ever stop taking your medication without first consulting your doctor.*

Your relationship with your doctor is critical. In choosing a doctor, get referrals from friends and other physicians, ask questions, and be an informed consumer. The responsibility for managing your hypertension is a partnership. Ask questions of the doctor and insist on explantions you can understand. The fact that you are reading a book about your disease is a good beginning. When you go to your doctor have a list of questions written down. This lets the doctor know you

---

Patient Guidelines for Hypertension Drug Therapy

Dr. Randall M. Zusman, director of the Hypertension Clinic at Massachusetts General Hospital, issues these guidelines for his patients on drug therapy.

To help you achieve better blood pressure control, try following these general guidelines:

1. An important part of blood pressure control is unrelated to your medications; it is important that you:

Stop smoking.

Avoid salt (do not add salt to your food; if possible, avoid all high–salt-containing foods).

Lose weight (if you're overweight).

Exercise regularly.

2. Take your medications as prescribed at the same time every day.

3. *Never increase, decrease, stop, or start* your medications on your own; doing so could be extremely dangerous; contact your doctor if you think your medication should be changed.

4. If another doctor changes your blood pressure medication for any reason, ask him or her to send a letter to your hypertension doctor (the physician who has diagnosed your high blood pressure and prescribed treatment) explaining what change was made and why.

5. Ask that copies of any blood tests you have undergone, X rays, or any other tests including EKGs, be sent to your hypertension doctor.

6. Take advantage of every opportunity to have your blood pressure measured by a health-care professional (not by a machine—many times this testing is offered for free as a community service in shopping malls, at street fairs, or in your office); record all blood pressure measurements and bring them to your next appointment.

7. Don't run out of medication; *suddenly stopping your pills can be extremely dangerous*—if you need a prescription, call the office before running out of medication and be sure to ask for new prescriptions during your office visits to avoid running out of pills.

8. If you are hospitalized for any reason, be sure that your hypertension doctor is informed. Also be sure to tell the admitting doctor at the hospital you have high blood pressure and what medicines you are taking.

9. Keep a list of all the names of your medicines and the exact doses in your wallet so you can be specific about this information.

are interested in finding out about your condition, respect the doctor's time, and want to participate in your care. Ask about alternative treatments, side effects, cost, and prognosis. Be sure you understand the responses before you leave the office.

Antihypertensive Drug Therapy

The goals of drug therapy to control hypertension are to

- Control blood pressure.
- Maintain well-being.
- Prevent end organ complications.
- Reduce cardiovascular risks.

These are also the goals of preventing high blood pressure in the first place if it runs in your family.

If the decision is made to put you on medication, a series of other choices have to be made. In the past few decades, great strides have been made in the development of antihypertensive drugs and a wide range of treatments now exist, each of which can be tailored to your specific needs. Basically, however, the drugs work within your system to lower blood pressure in three different ways:

- A medicine can interfere with the ability of the sympathetic nervous system to transmit messages to the blood pressure "machines"—the heart, kidney, and adrenal glands.
- A medicine can interfere with the ability of a blood pressure machine to receive the message to raise the

blood pressure, even though it gets out of the *sympathetic nervous system.*

- A medicine can force one of the blood pressure machines to obey *its* orders rather than those of the sympathetic nervous system.

Which of these three mechanisms, each of which works on a different part of the blood pressure control system, should be used to treat your particular case of hypertension? In choosing a drug therapy, your doctor will take into consideration a number of factors: the possible side effects of the drugs, how well you respond to taking the drugs, if more than one drug is needed, and other conditions or disorders you might have along with your hypertension.

What do you need to know about the medicines that you are taking? You need to know which machine in the blood pressure control system they affect—the heart, kidney, or adrenal glands—so that you can be aware of what is happening to your body and what side effects to expect. You need to know what over-the-counter medicines might interfere with your hypertensive medications. And if you're pregnant or nursing, you need to know if a medicine will be harmful to you or your baby.

Four classes of drugs work to lower high blood pressure: (1) *diuretics* cause the kidney to excrete more sodium and fluid; (2) *antiadrenergic agents* act to block sympathetic nervous system signals from being sent or received by the other blood pressure organs; (3) *vasodilators* force artery walls to dilate, thereby decreasing pressure; and (4) *angiotensin-converting enzyme (ACE) inhibitors* prevent the secretion of angiotensin II, the hormone that acts both to constrict blood vessels and to stimulate the adrenal glands, which cause the kidney to absorb more sodium and fluid.

Within each class of drugs, there are a number of different medicines, each of which acts in a slightly different way from the others. A complete discussion of these drugs goes far beyond the scope of this chapter; please consult your physician and/or one of the many books that deal specifically with blood pressure drug therapy (see chapter 8). The following descriptions of the drug classes will give you a general overview of both side effects and benefits so that you can discuss options with your physician.

The Diuretics. Medicines that reduce the volume of the body's blood and fluids, known as diuretics, were first developed in the late 1950s. This group of drugs lowers blood pressure by increasing the kidney's excretion of sodium and water. Treatment with diuretics can cause about a 2-quart reduction in a patient's fluid volume; this lower volume lessens both heart action and pressure on the vessel walls.

Today, three types of diuretics are used. The most common diuretics are the *thiazides,* which block the reabsorption of sodium and chloride back into the bloodstream. Thiazides are the most frequently used and most extensively investigated of the diuretics and are usually the drug of first choice for most patients with mild to moderate hypertension.

Loop diuretics are stronger drugs, usually reserved

for patients whose blood pressure is not adequately lowered by the thiazide or who have damaged kidneys. Loop diuretics, so named because they work in the part of the kidney known as Henle's loop, are quite potent; in fact they eliminate about 15 percent more salt from the kidneys than do the thiazides.

The third type of diuretic includes the *potassium-sparing agents*. This class of drugs was developed when physicians discovered that, along with the sodium, diuretics eliminated another important mineral, potassium. Potassium is essential for proper muscle function, and that includes heart action. When potassium loss does occur, patients experience a number of dangerous side effects, including irregular heartbeat, muscle weakness, kidney malfunction, and often, glucose intolerance, which may trigger or exacerbate diabetes mellitus. Potassium depletion is referred to as hypokalemia. Potassium-sparing diuretics work in the exchange sites of the kidneys to increase sodium excretion while maintaining potassium levels. They are usually used in conjunction with other diuretics to compensate for the potential loss of potassium.

In recent years, increasing resistance to the routine use of diuretics has occurred, primarily because of the wide-ranging, often severe side effects. Prolonged use of diuretics often causes an increase in circulating cholesterol and other lipids, which adds to the risk of stroke from atherosclerosis; they may also exacerbate diabetes. If you are predisposed to any of these disorders, that predisposition should be discussed with your physician as part of the decision on the use of diuretics to lower your blood pressure.

The Antiadrenergic Agents. Without any conscious effort, a part of our nervous system, the *sympathetic nervous system,* works to keep our internal environment stable and constant. One part of the sympathetic nervous system's job is to speed up the heart and constrict the blood vessels when signaled by the release of the stress hormones, which include norepinephrine and epinephrine.

As we learned in chapter 2, these two hormones, secreted by the kidneys, act as messengers between the sympathetic nervous system and the heart, blood vessels, and kidneys. One way antiadrenergic agents work is to keep these two substances from delivering the messages by blocking the nerve cells on the surface of vessel walls and within the heart and kidney. Another way is to prevent the message from ever leaving the brain in the first place. Five types of antiadrenergic drugs work on different parts of the sympathetic nervous system to reduce blood pressure.

Central-acting drugs lower blood pressure by stimulating certain nerve receptors, located in the brain itself, which act to reduce the heart rate, the amount of blood pumped by the heart, and the resistance of the blood vessels. The most common drugs in this category include methyldopa, clonidine, guanabenz, and guanfacine.

Peripheral inhibitors interfere with the release of norepinephrine from sympathetic nerve endings. Without norepinephrine, vessel walls will not contract and blood pressure will not rise. Reserpine is the most popular of the peripheral inhibitors, usually prescribed in conjunction with a diuretic. In fact, sodium and water retention is a common side effect of these drugs if a diuretic is not taken.

Alpha-blockers are designed to lower blood pressure by dilating the arteries and arterioles. An important element of alpha-blockers is that they do not decrease heart action. This makes them especially useful for treating younger, more active patients who want to exercise at or near their maximum heart rate. In addition, alpha-blockers often raise the level of HDLs (the "good" cholesterol) while lowering total lipid levels, a boon to patients who have atherosclerosis. Doctors prescribe the alpha-blockers prazosin and terazosin most often.

Next to diuretics, *beta-blockers* are the most commonly prescribed antihypertensive medications with more than 30 million prescriptions nationwide. Beta-blockers work in two ways. First, they inhibit the responses of the nerve cells in the heart, and second, they block the release of renin, the chemical secreted by the kidney that otherwise would initiate a chain reaction ending with increased heart rate and vessel contraction.

Beta-blockers are particularly useful when prescribed in conjunction with vasodilators and diuretics, although about half of all patients with mild hypertension can be treated with beta-blockers alone. These drugs, which include metaproterenol, atenolol, nadolol, and others, are especially useful for patients who have had or run the risk of having a heart attack, because they considerably decrease heart action. Because of this effect, however, they are not recommended for those patients with a low heart rate (*bradycardia*) or congestive heart failure. In addition, athletes and other active patients may find the drugs' inhibiting effect on heart rate to be unacceptable.

It is important to keep in mind that all antiadrenergic drugs work to inhibit the nervous system in some way. Although this is quite effective in lowering blood pressure in most patients, these drugs also have a number of often disturbing side effects. Some patients, especially those who use beta-blockers, complain of lethargy, mild depression, impotence or lack of sexual desire, and respiratory problems. These symptoms result from the fact that your responses to stimuli are, in effect, dulled by this type of medication. Although many physicians and patients alike feel that the benefits of treatment with antiadrenergic drugs far outweigh such problems, you should be aware of these potential side effects and discuss them with your physician.

The Vasodilators. These drugs cause the smooth muscle of the vessel walls to relax, thereby allowing more blood to pass through the arteries with less resistance. While this does decrease blood pressure, it also stimulates the reaction of the other blood pressure control systems within the body. To compensate for this vessel dilation, the heart rate goes up, the kidneys retain more sodium and secrete more renin, and the adrenal glands release epinephrine and norepinephrine—all of which increase blood pressure. Thus concurrent treatment with other drugs is often necessary.

In general, vasodilators are reserved for older patients who have stiff vessel walls or for patients with severe hypertension. The most common vasodilators are hydralazine, minoxidil, and diazoxide.

The Angiotensin-Converting Enzyme Inhibitors. The newest of the antihypertensive drugs, the ACE inhibitors interrupt the chain reaction set off when the chemical renin is secreted by the kidney. As you may remember from chapter 2, when renin is produced, it releases the hormone angiotensin I, which is then converted by another enzyme into angiotensin II. Angiotensin II acts to raise the blood pressure in two ways: by constricting blood vessels and by stimulating the adrenal glands, which cause the kidneys to retain more sodium and fluid. Quite simply, the ACE inhibitors stop angiotensin I from being converted into angiotensin II, thus breaking this blood pressure raising chain.

These drugs are unique among blood pressure medications in that as well as preventing the vessels from constricting, they also tend to help the body excrete sodium and fluid. Another positive characteristic of these drugs is that they help the kidneys retain potassium, thereby eliminating the need for a potassium-sparing agent. Especially useful for hypertensive diabetics and those with atherosclerosis, ACE inhibitors rarely raise glucose or blood lipid levels as do many other medications.

The Calcium Channel Blockers. Calcium channel blockers work to relax vascular smooth muscle in a slightly different way from vasodilators. Calcium, a vital chemical, has a major influence on muscle contraction. By varying the concentration of calcium in the cells, muscles can be made to either contract or relax.

Calcium channel blockers lessen the availability of calcium to the cells in the arterial walls, causing them to relax, thus allowing the blood pressure to go down.

These drugs also affect heart action. The speed with which your heart beats is controlled by a mass of specialized tissue, called the *pacer,* located in the right atrium. The action of the pacer is also affected by calcium. When a calcium channel blocker is used, the heart rate is lowered.

Calcium channel blockers, which include verapamil, diltiazem, and nifedipine, are now often the first choice medications, because they are generally quite safe, well tolerated, and cause a minimum of side effects. Unlike many other drugs, they do not cause salt retention in most patients, which relieves the need for a diuretic, although for people with moderate to severe hypertension the two types of drugs together can be quite effective. However, calcium channel blockers and beta-blockers, both of which reduce heart activity, should not be prescribed together.

The aim of drug therapy is to use the agents just described, alone or in combination, to lower arterial pressure to normal levels, with minimal side effects. In general, of course, the fewer pills and the fewer side effects, the better. As our knowledge of the underlying causes of hypertension grows, so too does our success rate in treating the disease with drugs. And as we learn more about what may be causing hypertension in individual patients, more patient-specific drug programs will become available. In the meantime, physicians try to match drug therapy with patient needs while limiting the number and amount of drugs as much as possible.

The Step-Care Approach

Except for those patients with severe hypertension, most patients are first treated with just one drug. Because many effective antihypertensive medicines are now available, a number of useful therapeutic regimens have been developed.

At one point, the step-care approach, suggested by the Joint National Committee on Detection, Evaluation, and Treatment of High Blood Pressure, was the primary approach. This program assumed that nearly all hypertensives should be treated similarly, and almost everyone started off with a thiazide diuretic. If that didn't work, other medicines were added in a fixed pattern until the blood pressure was normalized.

More treatment options are now available. The first choice is usually between one of the blockers and a diuretic. The reason for choosing one over the other varies from patient to patient. In general, African-Americans and the elderly will respond better to diuretics, and younger and Caucasian patients will respond better to either a beta-blocker or a calcium channel blocker.

In most cases of mild to moderate hypertension, one of the above drugs is prescribed alone at a relatively low dose. If that does not work on its own, another drug is added, at the same low dose. Alternatively, a higher dose of the first drug may be prescribed. This first phase of drug treatment usually lasts about eight weeks.

If combining low doses of a thiazide with a beta-blocker or calcium channel blocker does not reduce blood pressure to normal levels, then the blocker is increased to the full dose, which does the trick in most patients. Fewer than 5 percent of patients will still be hypertensive with this drug combination and dose. Very often a secondary cause of hypertension—kidney disease, aldosteronism, or Cushing's disease—is the culprit if the blood pressure has not been lowered.

If no secondary cause can be found, one of the other classes of antihypertensive drugs, either vasodilators or antiadrenergic agents, are added. At that point, once blood pressure is controlled, previous drugs are sequentially withdrawn to determine the minimum amount of drugs necessary.

While the recommendations outlined above work for most patients, it is important for physicians to use a flexible approach because individual patients may respond differently to different drugs and drug combinations. Every effort should be made to reduce the number of times each day the patient must interrupt his or her schedule for medication. Treatment for hypertension with drugs—if not combined with lifestyle changes that reduce risk factors—is usually lifelong, so it must be as easy and as side effect free as possible.

A general note of caution: When you take any medicine to treat high blood pressure, your blood pressure control system will be unable to respond to changes in posture as rapidly as it did before. All medicines used to treat high blood pressure, therefore, have a tendency to cause some light-headedness or dizziness when you sit, stand, or otherwise change your body position.

And, believe it or not, you may fall victim to *hypotension*—low blood pressure—while taking blood pressure medications, at least at first. Your blood pressure may lower quite rapidly, and your body will respond as if the blood pressure isn't normal: you may feel faint or dizzy or experience weakness in your arms and legs. Such symptoms should soon pass; however, if they persist, your doctor may prescribe another drug that will have fewer side effects.

Drug Therapy for Special Patients
Four groups of patients with hypertension require special consideration.

Kidney Disease Patients. If you have kidney disease, you may be one of the few patients with secondary hypertension, in which case you may need surgery (described later in this chapter) to correct your high blood pressure. In fact, many antihypertensive drugs directly affect kidney function and, therefore, may have adverse effects. If you have kidney disease, your physician will work with you to develop an appropriate treatment.

Heart Disease Patients. If you are taking medication for a heart condition, you should be aware that any decrease in potassium levels, common with the use of diuretics, is especially dangerous for you. Thiazide, therefore, should be used judiciously and a reduction in potassium should be corrected. Potassium replacement is frequently prescribed along with diuretic therapy. Calcium channel blockers and ACE inhibitors may be particularly useful for you; discuss them with your physician.

Diabetics. If you have diabetes as well as hypertension, finding drug therapy that works for you may be tricky, because many of the drugs used to lower blood pressure can exacerbate diabetes. Your doctor may prescribe ACE inhibitors for you, because they have no known adverse effects on glucose or lipid levels. They may actually minimize the development of diabetes-related kidney disease by relaxing blood vessels in the kidney.

Pregnant Women. If you are pregnant and have high blood pressure or if you develop hypertension during your pregnancy, you must be particularly careful about drug therapy. You have to be sure that while reducing your own blood pressure, the blood pressure of the fetus is kept at a normal level. In fact, during the second and third trimesters, antihypertensive medication is not indicated for any pregnant woman unless the diastolic pressure exceeds 95 millimeters of mercury. Diuretics and beta-blockers are often not prescribed because they may endanger the fetus, but vasodilators have no known adverse effects on the fetus. Be certain to discuss all medical problems and medication with your obstetrician. Prenatal care is the key to a healthy baby. If your obstetrician changes your hypertension medication during your pregnancy, ask the doctor to coordinate this with the doctor in change of your hypertension medication.

Surgical Treatment of Hypertension

As we have discussed, more than 90 percent of all hypertensives have essential hypertension, for which no *one* cause or cure can be found. For those with essential hypertension, lifelong treatment with drug therapy and/or diet and exercise are the only methods available to treat their disease and, therefore, to prevent stroke and heart attack.

The other 10 percent of people with high blood pressure can trace the cause of their disease to a specific physiological defect. If someone with hypertension fails to respond to standard drug therapy or exhibits certain symptoms, a doctor will go beyond the standard urine and blood tests to determine if the patient has one of these specific conditions. Secondary hypertensives quite often require surgery to correct their condition, and once the surgery is performed, blood pressure usually returns to normal, or at least is much easier to control.

Kidney Disorders

Renal artery stenosis is a condition in which the large artery that brings blood to the kidneys is narrowed or blocked. The approach in most cases is to repair or bypass the blockage of the artery so that blood supply to the kidney is restored. Another technique, called *percutaneous transluminal angioplasty,* involves inserting a small balloon into the artery with a needle, then inflating the balloon to widen the vessel. Although this method of correcting renal artery stenosis is uncommon, it does alleviate the need for major surgery in some patients.

Unfortunately, if the renal artery is blocked as a result of atherosclerosis, there's a good chance that *renal small vessel disease* is also present—the tiny arterioles and capillaries within the kidney are also narrowed by fatty plaque. In this case, surgery on the renal artery is less successful, because it will not completely solve the underlying problem of atherosclerosis throughout the kidney. The surgery does, however, often improve the kidney blood flow. This makes future drug therapy easier, and in some cases improves kidney function.

Endocrine Disorders

A rare condition known as *hyperaldosteronism* causes hypertension when a tumor on one or both adrenal glands causes the release of too much aldosterone. The hormone aldosterone causes the kidneys to retain salt and water and to excrete potassium. Surgery to remove the tumor will often bring the blood pressure down to normal.

Cushing's disease is another rare abnormality of adrenal gland function that causes hypertension. The adrenal glands of patients with Cushing's disease produce too much cortisol, a hormone that helps regulate metabolism. Hypertension is only one symptom of this often devastating disease. Overproduction of cortisol causes dramatic weight gain, fatigue, cessation of menstruation, skin changes, and even alterations in personality. Surgery to correct whatever is causing the adrenal glands to malfunction usually cures this disease.

Pheochromocytoma is an extremely rare disease in which a tumor causes part of the sympathetic nervous system to manufacture too much norepinephrine and epinephrine. Again, surgery to remove the tumor causing the problem is often the only way to reduce high blood pressure in these patients. This disorder occasionally runs in families and is passed along genetically. It may be associated with other endocrine abnormalities.

Keep in mind that it is highly unlikely that your high blood pressure is being caused by one of these uncommon disorders. If you have not responded to persistent drug therapy and/or lifestyle modification, ask your doctor if you should be screened for one of the above diseases.

It is up to you and your doctor to find a way—through a good deal of cooperation and communication—to lower your blood pressure. Remember you are both working to prevent damage to your circulatory system.

Questions and Answers

Q: I'm forty years old, have a family history of hypertension and stroke, and have a blood pressure of 170/100 millimeters of mercury. My doctor wants to put me on medication, but I'm afraid that if I start taking these drugs, I'll never be able to stop taking them—and I don't want to have to take drugs for the rest of my life. I have about 20 pounds to lose, and I just stopped smoking. Could I solve my problem without drugs?

A: In the long run, you might be able to control your hypertension without medication. However, right now your blood pressure is in the danger zone for someone with your family history of stroke. With the addition of your weight problem and history of smoking, your doctor is probably right to put you on medication immediately.

It is possible that once your blood pressure is controlled and you've lost the weight, lowered your fat and salt intake, and perhaps started and/or maintained an exercise program, your doctor may slowly take you off the antihypertensive medication. However, *do not* stop taking your medication without first consulting your physician.

Q: I'm a thirty-six-year-old new mother who developed high blood pressure during my pregnancy. I want to nurse, but am afraid the drugs I've been prescribed will harm my baby. Are there any high blood pressure medicines that I can use?

A: This is a tricky question, because almost every medicine taken enters breast milk to some degree, and that is equally true for blood pressure medications. Some drugs enter the breast milk freely, others in very limited amounts. The American Academy of Pediatrics considers alpha- and beta-blockers to be safe for breast-feeding mothers, but discourages the use of thiazide diuretics, because they can suppress the milk supply. If you have mild hypertension, you may want to discuss with your doctor nondrug therapy, at least until you stop nursing your baby.

Q: I've just started to take medication for high blood pressure. I frequently feel dizzy—sometimes almost to the point of fainting—when I stand up. I also feel lethargic and a little depressed. In fact, I feel sicker now than before I started to take medication. Is my condition getting worse or are these side effects of the drugs?

A: Although dizziness may also be a sign of severe high blood pressure, the symptoms you describe are most likely side effects of antihypertension drug therapy. The drugs used to treat high blood pressure are powerful and often act on your nervous system in ways that not only lower arterial pressure but also produce unpleasant side effects. Some symptoms, especially dizziness, may subside once your body adjusts to the medicine. If the symptoms persist for more than a week or so, speak to your physician. Other drugs, of which there are literally dozens, may better suit your particular body chemistry.

Caution: Do not stop taking your medication without consulting your doctor. If left untreated, high blood pressure may cause serious and often fatal damage to your circulatory system.

Q: My doctor tells me that my hypertension is caused by renal artery stenosis—the large artery that brings blood to the kidney is blocked. He says I need surgery to correct it. Can't my condition be treated with drug therapy?

A: Probably not, although drug therapy may still be necessary after the surgery. Surgery to correct renal artery stenosis usually involves removing the narrowed or blocked section of the artery so that the blood supply to the kidney is no longer compromised. Another method involves angioplasty, in which an instrument is advanced into the artery by a needle and a small balloon is inflated at the site of the blockage. The pressure exerted by the balloon forces the narrowed section to widen.

Once the obstruction is removed, blood pressure usually reverts to normal or near normal levels. However, most cases of renal artery stenosis are caused by atherosclerosis. If atherosclerosis is present in the main renal artery, it may well exist in small arteries of the kidney as well (a condition known as small vessel disease). Removing the obstruction will thus not solve the problem completely, and drug and diet therapy may be required. In some cases of advanced renal disease, surgery may not be recommended, because the risks will outweigh the benefits of surgery. Please discuss the matter thoroughly with your physician.

7

When Hypertension Is Uncontrolled

Six months have now passed since Angela's father experienced his cerebrovascular event and was warned about the dangers of high blood pressure and other risk factors. Although Charles has had no recurrences and appears and feels quite well, he remembers the incident vividly, as does his whole family. His children know how close he came to real tragedy and they fear for his future, as well as for their own. They've all been forced to confront the state of their own health, especially their own risks for hypertension that they may have inherited from their parents.

Despite the fact that Charles had for some time suffered a number of the risk factors for stroke—namely hypertension, diabetes, smoking, and a family history of hypertension—he never actually believed he'd be one of the more than 2 million people who are felled by a stroke or heart attack every year. In a way, none of us ever do believe it: strokes and heart attacks happen to other people—until it happens to us or to someone we love.

But with warning signs such as the one Charles and his family received, we have the opportunity to eliminate risk factors for both hypertension and the serious diseases it can cause.

The Effects of Hypertension

Hypertension and Atherosclerosis

Atherosclerosis is known as hypertension's deadly partner and for good reason: it is one of the most serious of all cardiovascular diseases; it is the leading cause of heart attack and stroke. While a certain degree of atherosclerosis is probably part of the natural aging process, hypertension is known to accelerate its development. Over a period of time, hypertension damages the walls of the arteries; the lesions that are formed from this damage become the focal point for the deposit of plaque.

As described in chapter 1, atherosclerosis occurs when deposits of fatty substances form on the wall of an artery. As the buildup thickens, arteries turn brittle and rough, losing their ability to expand and contract. If enough plaque accumulates, blood flow through the artery can become totally blocked.

When this happens, the tissues and organs supplied by the blood vessels are both deprived of nutrients and oxygen and prevented from releasing waste products into the bloodstream. When the heart fails to receive these vital elements and when waste products build up, the muscle becomes damaged and a heart attack ensues. If atherosclerosis blocks blood flow to the brain, a stroke occurs.

Hypertension and Stroke

The Brain. An extraordinarily complicated and intricate structure, the brain is host to millions of complex electrical and chemical actions and reactions taking place every second. How we think, what foods we like, how fast we run, who we love—all these functions and thousands more are stimulated by the brain and its intricate network of nerve cells distributed throughout the body.

The basic unit of your entire nervous system is the neuron, a tiny cell less than 1/100 of an inch in diameter. Your brain and nervous system consist of billions of neurons dispersed throughout the body and each of these cells require a constant supply of oxygen to function.

Stroke. Simply stated, a stroke occurs when the brain is deprived of its blood supply. Although stroke affects the brain, it is not technically a neurological disease. Basically, there are four principal types of stroke: two caused by clots and two, by hemorrhage. *Cerebral thrombosis* and *cerebral embolism,* which are caused by clots that plug one of the vessels in the brain, account for about 70 to 80 percent of all strokes.

Cerebral thrombosis is the most common type. It occurs when a blood clot forms in a major artery bringing blood to part of the brain. As we've seen, atherosclerosis is a major factor in the development of such cerebrovascular blockage, and hypertension is a major contributor to atherosclerosis.

A cerebral embolism is, in a way, a kind of traveling thrombus. It has the same effect as a thrombus—cutting off a portion of the brain's blood supply—but it originates in another part of the circulatory system and is brought to the site of the stroke through the bloodstream. Most emboli form when bits of atherosclerotic plaque in the carotid artery wall break off and get carried along in the bloodstream to the brain. An embolism can also be a clot that originates in the heart and is formed because the heart is beating irregularly (atrial fibrillation) or is damaged in another way. With either form of embolism, circulation to the brain tissue is damaged, resulting in a stroke.

Another type of stroke is caused by small vessel blockage within the brain itself. This results from hypertension and atherosclerosis. Vessels deep within the brain become blocked, cutting off the blood supply to small areas of the brain. Called *lacunar strokes,* the cerebrovascular events that result from small vessel disease account for approximately 10 percent of all strokes.

About 5 to 10 percent of strokes are caused when a diseased or damaged artery either in the brain or, less commonly, in the tissue that surrounds the brain bursts. Called *cerebral hemorrhages,* these strokes are among the most lethal because not only is the specific nerve tissue supplied by the damaged vessel injured but the adjacent area is also deprived of blood. There are many different types of cerebral hemorrhage; where the hemorrhage takes place defines both the type and the amount of damage to the neurological system that results.

Just as hypertension is called the silent killer because of its lack of overt symptoms, strokes can also occur without warning. However, many patients are warned in advance that all is not well within their cardiovascular systems. They experience transient ischemic attacks (TIAs), which occur when a blood clot temporarily clogs an artery and part of the brain doesn't get the blood it needs to function properly.

A TIA is often called a ministroke. It is caused by *ischemia,* a blockage in one of the arteries feeding the brain. Once a TIA has occurred, it tends to recur unless the underlying cause is eliminated.

The symptoms of TIA include temporary weakness or paralysis on one side of the body, loss or impaired vision in one eye or difficulty in speaking—in short, all the trappings of a full-blown stroke, but without any lasting effects. TIAs are very strong predictors of stroke. Do not ignore them; see your physician immediately.

Hypertension and Heart Disease

The Heart. About the size of your fist, your heart is an amazingly resilient muscular organ. It beats an average of 72 times a minute, 100,000 times a day, resting just a fraction of a second between beats. It pumps your blood through more than 70,000 miles of blood vessels at the rate of 1 gallon a minute.

A normal adult circulatory system contains about 8 pints of blood, which is recirculated continuously throughout your body. A complete cycle, from the heart through the body and back again, takes just one minute. Without doubt, the heart works harder than any other muscle in the body.

Heart Disease and Heart Attacks. While a stroke is death of brain cells due to lack of oxygen, a heart attack is death of heart tissue due to lack of oxygen. When a combination of atherosclerosis and hypertension attack the arteries feeding the heart muscle, the condition is called *coronary heart disease.* The blood supply arteries become narrow or obstructed, preventing the heart from getting enough oxygen. When one or more of the coronary arteries become severely blocked, the heart is deprived of oxygen for long periods of time. This eventually leads to the irreversible damage and death of the portion of heart muscle supplied by that artery. The death of this tissue is called a heart attack, otherwise known as a *myocardial infarction.*

Like strokes, myocardial infarctions occur in a number of different ways. The enlarging plaque itself can cause critical narrowing of the artery, called *myocardial ischemia,* which can eventually cause irreversible damage to the heart muscle. A clot of blood or fat (known as a thrombus) can form in the narrowed portion of the artery or a clot formed elsewhere in the circulation can travel to the coronary artery, where it then effectively shuts off the oxygen supply. This type of heart attack is called a *coronary embolism.*

Another form of heart disease caused primarily by hypertension occurs because the heart is forced to pump even harder to force the blood through narrowed arteries. Over time, this extra work actually causes the heart to enlarge. It becomes thicker and wider because of the additional stress and the larger volume of fluid it is forced to accommodate. The muscle tissue is damaged and the heart no longer pumps efficiently. Eventually, the enlarged heart may lose its capacity to push blood out of its chambers; fluid builds up and is forced back into the lungs. This results in *congestive heart failure*. Congestive heart failure can also occur after a myocardial infarction if enough muscle tissue has been damaged.

Like stroke, the heart attack is often proceeded by a warning sign, known in this case as *angina*. Angina is a transient chest pain due to lack of oxygen from the diminished blood supply to the heart muscle. Like stroke's TIA, angina causes symptoms similar to what would be experienced in a full-blown heart attack: a sensation of pain and tightening in the chest, heavy pressure or pain behind the breastbone, and pain that radiates to the neck, shoulder, arm, hands, or back. The patient experiencing angina may experience a feeling of strangling and anxiety as did Charles. Angina is often a sign that a serious problem exists with the oxygen supply to the heart muscle. If you experience chest pain at any time, see your doctor immediately.

Hypertension and Kidney Disease

The Kidneys. As you read in chapter 4, the kidneys are a pair of bean-shaped organs that lie at the base of the abdominal cavity. Each kidney is only about 4 inches long, 2 inches wide, and 1 inch thick and weighs only 5 to 6 ounces. Yet this amazing organ receives about one-quarter of the volume of every heartbeat—about 1.5 quarts of blood per minute. The arrangement of vessels necessary to control and handle this task is quite complex.

The kidney's functioning unit is called the nephron, which are cuplike receptacles. There are about 1 million nephrons per kidney. Each of these long tubular units empties the blood entering the kidney into the center of the organ, where waste products are separated and eliminated from our bodies through the production of urine. By eliminating waste, the kidneys regulate the level of fluid in the body, including the blood.

In addition, the kidneys play another integral role in the blood pressure system. Each nephron is also equipped with a group of specialized cells that release certain chemical messengers, or hormones, to control the blood pressure in the body. If these cells sense that the pressure is too low, the messenger causes the muscles in the walls of all the vessels in the body to contract, raising the blood pressure. If the pressure is too high, less of the hormone is made and the vessels tend to relax. Another message may be sent to another part of the kidney to either retain more salt and water, raising the pressure, or to excrete more salt and water, thereby lowering pressure.

Kidney Disease. When the arteries and tiny vessels feeding the kidney become clogged by plaque due to hypertension and atherosclerosis, a condition known as *nephrosclerosis* occurs. The result is that the kidney loses its ability to filter waste products out of the body.

Kidney failure results when the kidneys begin to lose their filtering function. Most patients have no symptoms until they start to retain large amounts of fluid. This leads to higher blood pressure. The kidneys can only withstand so much pressure and stress before they fail. Diabetes creates another situation that damages the kidneys. The cycle of damaged kidneys, hypertension, and kidney failure is common.

Hypertension and Your Eyes

Another result of high blood pressure is reduced vision, even blindness. This occurs when blood vessels in the eyes rupture because of the stress of the high arterial pressure. This is especially frequent in diabetics.

Living Life Hypertension Free

Take another look at the risk factors, controllable and uncontrollable, listed in chapter 1. Are you at risk? If so, the resources given in chapter 8 will help you learn more about the proven ways of reducing risk for hypertension, including regulating diet, exercising, stopping smoking, reducing stress, and undergoing drug and surgical therapies.

Take advantage of these resources. Many of these organizations offer free materials and advice, and many of them have branch offices throughout the country. And, if you should need more information than they offer, they'll be able to recommend the agency or organization that can best help you.

8

Resources

The American Heart Association

The American Heart Association, with branches in every major city across the country, offers information about all aspects of cardiovascular disease. Diet and exercise plans to lower blood pressure; research papers describing the latest medical breakthroughs in diagnosis and treatment; and pamphlets describing symptoms of heart disease, strokes, and other cardiovascular ailments are available through this organization.

The American Heart Association
7320 Greenville Avenue
Dallas, TX 75231
(214) 373–6300

Other Organizations

American Medical Association
535 North Dearborn Street
Chicago, IL 60610
(312) 464–5000

**Heart and Stroke Foundation
of Canada**
160 George Street
Suite 200
Ottawa, Ont. K1N9M2
(613) 237–4361

**The National Easter Seal
Society**
2023 West Ogden Avenue
Chicago, IL 60612
(312) 726–6200

General Information

General information on prevention and treatment of hypertension and other cardiovascular disease is available from the American Red Cross and the Office of Disease Prevention. In addition, should you want to learn more about cardiopulmonary resuscitation (CPR) and other emergency care procedures, the Red Cross offers classes in many communities. Please note that there are branches of the Red Cross in major cities across the country.

American Red Cross
Seventeenth and D Streets
NW
Washington, DC 20006
(301) 737–8300

**Office of Disease Prevention
and Health Promotion**
National Health Information
Center
P.O. Box 1133
Washington, DC 20013-
11332
(301) 565–4167
(800) 565–4797

Exercise

Physical fitness is a sure-fire way to reduce hypertension and the risk for stroke. In almost every town in the country, health clubs and spas, not to mention the local YMCA, can help you get in shape. In addition to those organizations, you can contact the following groups:

American Alliance for Health, Physical Education, and Recreation
1201 Sixteenth Street NW
Washington, DC 20036

The President's Council on Physical Fitness and Sports
400 Sixth Street NW
Washington, DC 20201
(202) 272–3430

Quitting Smoking

Many people need encouragement and help to stop smoking. The organizations listed below can give you advice on how to stop smoking on your own or recommend reputable medical or psychological techniques.

American Cancer Society
National Office
19 West Fifty-sixth Street
New York, NY 10001
(212) 586–8700

Canadian Cancer Society
77 Bloor Street
Suite 1701
Toronto, Ont. M5S3A1
(416) 961–7223

American Lung Association
1740 Broadway
New York, NY 10019
(212) 315–8700

National Cancer Institute
Office of Cancer
Communications
Bethesda, MD 20205
(301) 496–4000

For Diabetics

Diabetes is one of hypertension's deadliest associates and, combined with smoking and atherosclerosis, is a leading risk factor in the development of stroke and heart attacks. For more information on treatment for diabetes, contact the following organizations.

American Diabetes Association, Inc.
2 Park Avenue
New York, NY 10016
(212) 947–9707

The Juvenile Diabetes Foundation
60 Madison Avenue
New York, NY 10017
(212) 689–2860

Institute of Diabetes and Digestive Diseases
9000 Rockville Pike
Bethesda, MD 20892
(301) 496–3583

National Diabetes Association
78 Bond Street
Toronto, Ont. M5B2JH
(416) 362–4440

Eye Care

One of the most unfortunate side effects of hypertension—as well as diabetes and other diseases related to aging—is vision impairment. If your eyesight has been affected by one of these conditions, the following organizations can provide you with help.

American Academy of Ophthalmology
P.O. Box 7424
San Francisco, CA 94120-7424
(415) 561–8500

National Society to Prevent Blindness
500 East Remington Road
Schaumburg, IL 60173
(708) 843–2020

Kidney Disease

Damage to the kidneys is both a cause and an effect of high blood pressure. The National Kidney Foundation is an excellent source of general information about all aspects of kidney disease. For patients who have specific kidney problems and want to learn more about support groups for kidney patients or receive the quarterly publication *Renal Life*, written by and for people with kidney disorders, contact the American Association of Kidney Patients.

American Association of
Kidney Patients
1 Davis Boulevard
Suite LLI
Tampa, FL 33606
(813) 251–0725

National Kidney Foundation
30 East Thirty-third Street
New York, NY 10016
(212) 889–2210

Stroke and Its Aftermath

For many stroke survivors and their families, the feelings of isolation and loneliness are the toughest after-effects of stroke. Fortunately, support groups, called stroke clubs, have been set up all over the country to lend friendship, mutual assistance, and fellowship.

Often stroke clubs are sponsored by local hospitals or local chapters of the National Easter Seal Society and the American Heart Association (addresses given above). In addition, the National Stroke Association, an organization started in 1984 to concentrate on prevention of stroke and the treatment and rehabilitation of the stroke survivor, is developing a national listing of all stroke clubs across the country. For further information about stroke prevention and treatment, the National Stroke Association has an extensive list of publications and videos. Write to them for a publications list, as well as for information about a stroke club near your home.

National Institute of Neurological Disorders and Stroke
9000 Rockville Pike
Bethesda, MD 20892
(301) 496–5751

The National Stroke
Association
1565 Clarkson Street
Denver, CO 80218
(303) 839–1992

Information for the Older Patient

National and state agencies on aging can help you with any questions you may have about Medicare; home nursing care; and many other issues associated with aging, illness, and stroke in particular. Check your telephone directory for local agencies or contact the following national organization for assistance.

Medicaid/Medicare
Health Financing Administration
Department of Health and Human Services
Washington, DC 20201
(202) 245–0312

For Additional Reading

There have been a number of excellent books published on hypertension, stroke, and heart disease, many of which will help you learn about the causes and effects of high blood pressure, how stroke affects the brain and the body, and recuperation after a stroke. A partial list follows.

American Heart Association. *Heartbook: A Guide to Prevention and Treatment of Cardiovascular Diseases.* New York: E. P. Dutton, 1980.

Kenneth H. Cooper. *Overcoming Hypertension.* New York: Bantam, 1990.

Peggy Jo Donahue. *How to Prevent a Stroke.* Emmaus, Pa.: Rodale Press, 1989.

Ruth Esheleman and Mary Winston, compilers. *The American Heart Association Cookbook.* New York: Ballantine Books, 1987.

Conn Foley and H. F. Pizer. *The Stroke Fact Book.* New York: Bantam, 1985.

Norman M. Kaplan. *Clinical Hypertension,* 4th ed. Baltimore: Williams & Wilkins, 1986.

Norman M. Kaplan. *Management of Hypertension,* 2nd ed. Durant, Okla.: Creative Infomatics, Inc., 1987.

Richard D. Moore and George D. Webb. *The K Factor: Reversing and Preventing High Blood Pressure without Drugs.* New York: Macmillan, 1986.

Dean Ornish. *Program for Reversing Heart Disease.* New York: Random House, 1990.

Michael K. Rees. *The Complete Guide to Living with High Blood Pressure.* New York: Prentice Hall, 1988.

James V. Warren and Genell J. Subak-Sharpe. *Managing Hypertension.* New York: Doubleday, 1986.

Glossary

Agnosia. A perceptual impairment resulting in the inability to recognize familiar objects perceived by the senses or to associate an object with its use.

Aldosterone. A *steroid** hormone that is released by the adrenal gland and acts on the *kidney* to promote conservation of *sodium* and water, thereby raising blood pressure.

Alpha-blockers. Antihypertensive drugs that lower blood pressure by working with the *autonomic nervous system* to dilate the *blood vessels*.

Aneurysm. A weakened portion of a *blood vessel* wall that swells outward like a balloon. Factors that contribute to their formation are age, hypertension, atherosclerosis, and heredity. Aneurysms are found on tiny *arteries* within the brains of elderly and hypertensive patients. These aneurysms may rupture, causing *cerebral hemorrhage*.

*Italicized words have their own entry in the glossary.

Angiotensin. A substance in the blood produced in response to release of the enzyme *renin* by the *kidneys*. Angiotensin is an important *vasoconstrictor*. Angiotensin also causes an increase in the output of *aldosterone*.

Aorta. The main artery in the body, from which all others branch; the principal *blood vessel* leading away from the heart.

Aphasia. The inability to speak or understand spoken language. It is caused by an injury to the dominant sphere of the brain. This is the left side of the brain in a right-handed individual. The left-brain is dominant in two-thirds of left handers as well.

Arrhythmia. Irregular heartbeat that may be caused by heart disease but that also may occur without known cause. It can result in acutely lowered blood pressure, stroke, heart attack, or death.

Arachnoid. The middle of the three membranes covering the brain and spinal cord. Between it and the brain itself lies the subarachnoid space, which contains large blood vessels. See *Subarachnoid hemorrhage.*

Arteries. *Blood vessels* that carry blood and oxygen away from the heart to nourish cells throughout the body. The walls consist of muscle, which contracts or dilates to raise or lower blood pressure.

Arteriogram. An examination of a portion of the circulatory system performed by injecting dye through a catheter into the *arteries* thereby forming a map of the *blood vessels.*

Arterioles. Small arterial *blood vessels* most responsible for the control of blood pressure. They pass blood from the *arteries* to the *capillaries.*

Aspirin. A drug (acetylsalicylic acid) that reduces inflammation and fever. It is also known to affect the adhesiveness of *platelets* in the blood. This action is thought to reduce atherosclerosis.

Ataxia. A lack of coordination, unsteady gait, and poor balance usually resulting from stroke but may be the result of heredity or other birth defects.

Atherosclerosis. A disease of the *arteries* in which fatty plaques develop on the inner walls. This condition raises blood pressure and sets the stage for *thrombosis*.

Atrium. Two upper chambers of the heart.

Autonomic nervous system. The part of the *nervous system* that is responsible for bodily functions not consciously directed, such as the heartbeat, digestion, salivation, and so on. It is the autonomic nervous system that works to control the blood pressure. It is divided into two separate divisions: the *sympathetic nervous system* and the *parasympathetic nervous system*.

Baroreceptors. Nerve cells that monitor changes in blood pressure. The main receptors are the *carotid sinus* and the aortic arch. Impulses from the baroreceptors are sent to the *medulla oblongata*, the center of the *autonomic nervous system*.

Basilar artery. The artery at the base of the brain formed by the joining of the two *vertebral arteries*. The basilar arteries nourish the *hindbrain* with oxygen- and nutrient-rich blood.

Beta-blocker. A drug that prevents stimulation of certain receptors of the nerves of the *sympathetic ner-*

vous system, which would otherwise increase the heart rate.

Biofeedback. A behavior-modification therapy in which patients are taught to control usually unconscious bodily functions such as blood pressure through conscious effort. In addition, biofeedback is used as a stroke rehabilitation method.

Blood-brain barrier. The theoretical membrane that separates circulating blood from the tissue fluids that surround the brain cells, protecting the brain from solid particles and large molecules.

Blood vessel. Tubes of *smooth muscle* that carry blood to and from the heart. *Arteries* and *veins* are the two main types of blood vessels.

Bradycardia. Abnormally low heart rate; when the heart beats less than fifty times per minute. This can result in dangerously lowered blood pressure.

Brain stem. The lower part of the brain extension within the skull, consisting of the *medulla oblongata,* the *pons,* and the *midbrain.* The brain stem is a center for the regulation of breathing, heart action, and facial movement. When a *stroke* occurs in the brain stem, it is usually fatal.

Bruit. The noise blood makes when passing through *blood vessels* damaged by *atherosclerosis* or other diseases or conditions that cause turbulence in the vessels.

Caffeine. An alkaloid drug that stimulates the *central nervous system.* Most often found in coffee, tea, and many cola-based soft drinks.

Calcium channel blockers. Drugs that keep some calcium from reaching the vascular *smooth muscles*, thereby dilating the *blood vessels*, lowering arterial pressure.

Capillaries. The smallest of the *blood vessels*; they form networks in most *tissues*. Their blood is supplied by *arterioles*, and their walls are just one cell thick, which allows fluids, oxygen, and other nutrients to pass through to the various body *tissues*.

Carbohydrates. Organic compounds of carbon, hydrogen, and oxygen that represent an important part of our diet. They include starches, cellulose, and sugars and are an important source of energy. All carbohydrates are eventually broken down in the body into *glucose*. Excess carbohydrates are stored as *fats* in the liver and muscles.

Cardiac muscle. The muscle walls of the heart.

Cardiovascular system. The heart together with the two networks of *blood vessels* (*arteries* and *veins*) transport nutrients and oxygen to the *tissues* and remove waste products.

Carotid arteries. Two main *arteries* supply blood to the head and neck; one is set on each side of the skull. Each has two branches, internal and external. The internal carotid artery supplies the brain and the external carotid artery sends blood to the face, scalp, and neck. The branch point between internal and external is called the carotid bulb. It is a frequent location for atherosclerosis.

Carotid sinus. An area of the *carotid artery*, located at its division in the neck. Special nerve cells sense any changes in blood pressure and respond by changing the heart rate.

Catheterization. A procedure in which a small flexible tube is inserted into the body for the process of diagnosis or treatment, as in an *arteriogram*.

Central nervous system. The brain and the spinal cord, which are responsible for the integration of all neurologic functions.

Cerebellum. The largest part of the hindbrain located behind the *pons* and the *medulla oblongata*. It is responsible for movement coordination, muscle tone, and balance.

Cerebrum. The largest part of the brain; it controls thinking, the emotions, and voluntary activities. It consists of two halves (the cerebral hemispheres), which are joined together.

Cerebral cortex. The part of the brain most directly responsible for consciousness, perception, memory, thought, intellect, and all voluntary movement.

Cerebral edema. Swelling of brain tissue.

Cerebral hemorrhage. Bleeding from an artery that has ruptured into or around the brain. The vessel may be abnormal due to congenital causes or damaged by disease, including hypertension.

Cerebral thrombosis. The blockage of an artery supplying part of the brain with blood.

Cerebrovascular accident. See *stroke*.

Cholesterol. A fatlike substance found in the brain, nerves, liver, blood, and bile. Synthesized in the liver, cholesterol is essential for a number of bodily functions. Excess consumption of dietary cholesterol, found in animal products such as meats, whole milk, and eggs, contributes to *atherosclerosis* and coronary heart disease.

Chromosome. Any one of the tiny structures found in the nucleus of a cell that carries *heredity* information in the form of *genes*. There are forty-six chromosomes in each normal cell, twenty-three inherited from each parent.

Circle of willis. The connecting circle of *arteries* at the base of the brain into which branches of both *carotid* and *vertebral arteries* run; the means by which the blood supply to the brain is made more secure.

Coarctation of the aorta. A congenital narrowing of a short segment of the *aorta* between the upper and lower part of the body. Results in severe hypertension.

Coma. State of unconsciousness.

Collateral circulation. A rerouting of the blood through small vessels when a main *blood vessel* has been blocked by an embolus or thrombus.

Computer assisted tomography (CT) scan. An advanced form of X ray, which shows areas of the brain damaged by *stroke* or other injury.

Convulsion. Muscle *spasms* due to abnormal brain electrical stimulation.

Coronary arteries. The two vessels coming from the aorta to the heart. They go on to branch and supply the heart muscle with blood.

Coronary thrombosis. Blockage, by clotting, of one of the *coronary arteries* or one of the branches, especially by *atherosclerosis.*

Deoxyribonucleic acid (DNA). The fundamental component of all living matter, which controls and transmits the *genetic code.*

Diabetes mellitus. A chronic illness characterized by an excess of blood sugar due to either insufficient *insulin* production in the *pancreas* or the inability of the body to use insulin. Long-term effects of diabetes include increased risk for *atherosclerosis,* vision problems, kidney failure, and infections.

Diastole. The interval between heartbeats when the heart relaxes and fills with blood. The diastolic reading in a blood pressure measurement is the lower number.

Diuretic. A type of antihypertension drug that works to promote salt excretion by removing excess fluid.

Dysarthria. Speech impairment resulting from weakness in mouth, tongue, and jaw, causing slurring. See *aphasia.*

Edema. Abnormal swelling of body *tissue.*

Electrocardiography (EKG or ECG). A procedure in which heart function is measured by the tracing of its electrical impulses.

Electroencephalography (EEG). A procedure in which the electrical impulses from the brain are traced and recorded.

Embolism. Obstruction of a *blood vessel* by a blood clot or piece of plaque that has moved through the bloodstream from its point of origin to a narrower branch of the vessel. The material causing the resulting blockage is called an embolus. After the embolus has lodged in a vessel, that vessel can then clot off, resulting in *thrombosis*.

Endarterectomy. A surgical technique used to open an obstructed artery.

Endocrine system. A network of glands that secrete *hormones* into the bloodstream. Hormones control body processes, including digestion, circulation, reproduction, and growth, among many others.

Epinephrine. Also called adrenaline. A hormone secreted by the adrenal glands, situated just above the *kidneys*. Increases the body's capacity to respond in stressful conditions by increasing heart rate and constricting certain *blood vessels*.

Essential hypertension. High blood pressure caused by an unknown factor or factors. Accounts for approximately 90 percent of *hypertension* cases. See *secondary hypertension*.

Fat. An essential nutrient. The principal form in which energy is stored in the body.

Fibrillation. Uncoordinated tremors of the heart resulting in an irregular pulse. Atrial fibrillation is caused by *atherosclerosis* and hypertension.

Fight or flight response. The body's response to perceived danger or stress, involving the release of hormones and subsequent rise in heart rate, blood pressure, and muscle tension.

First-degree relative. A relative within your immediate family unit: parents, siblings, and offspring.

Ganglion. One of a group of nerve cells located outside

the brain and spinal cord. The ganglion acts as a control or switching center.

Gene. The part of the *chromosome* that determines *hereditary* characteristics.

Genetic code. The information carried by DNA (*deoxyribonucleic acid*) within each cell that determines *heredity*.

Gland. Any organ that produces and secretes a chemical substance for use by another part of the body.

Glucose. The most common simple sugar; essential source of energy for the body. It is stored in the liver as glycogen but can be converted back into glucose rapidly.

Glucose tolerance test. A diagnostic test for the presence of *diabetes mellitus*.

Heart attack. *Myocardial infarction.* Damage to the heart caused by interruption of the blood circulation through the *coronary arteries*.

Hemianopsia. Damage to the optic nerve, caused by brain damage, which results in blindness in one-half of each eye. It may be temporary or permanent.

Hemiplegia. Paralysis of one side of the body caused by brain injury. It may be temporary as in a TIA or permanent as in a stroke.

Hemisphere. One of the two halves of the cerebrum.

Hemoglobin. The oxygen-carrying red pigment component of the red blood cells. Hemoglobin transports oxygen to the body *tissue* and removes carbon dioxide.

Hemorrhage. Bleeding due to the rupture of a *blood vessel.*

Heparin. A powerful anticoagulant found in the liver and other body *tissues* that acts to prevent clotting of the blood. It is also given therapeutically by injection.

Heredity. The transmission of physical, personality, and intellectual traits from parents to children. Genetic information is carried by the *chromosomes*.

Hindbrain. The back part of the brain comprising the *cerebellum, pons,* and *medulla oblongata* that is supplied with blood by the *vertebral arteries*.

Hormone. Body secretion that is transported by the bloodstream to various organs to regulate or modify vital bodily functions and processes.

Hyperaldosteronism. A form of *secondary hypertension* in which excessive amounts of the hormone *aldosterone* are secreted, setting off a chain of events that results in high blood pressure.

Hypercholesterolemia. Excess amounts of *cholesterol* in the blood due to a metabolic disorder in which the body manufactures too much or cannot process enough cholesterol.

Hyperlipidemia. An abnormally high concentration of *fats* in the bloodstream.

Hypertension. High blood pressure.

Hypokalemia. A depletion of potassium in the blood, which is a side effect of some antihypertension drugs.

Hypotension. Low blood pressure.

Infarction. The death of tissue that occurs when the blood supply to a localized part of the body is blocked.

Insulin. A *hormone* produced and secreted by the *pancreas*. Necessary for proper metabolism, particularly of *carbohydrates* and the uptake of *glucose*. It is given as injections in the treatment of diabetes.

Ischemia. Oxygen deficiency caused by an obstruction of the *blood vessel*.

Kidneys. The two bean-shaped glands, situated at the back of the abdomen, that regulate salt volume and composition of the body fluids by filtering the blood and eliminating waste through the production of urine.

Labile hypertension. One or more isolated high blood pressure readings. May indicate an increased risk of developing hypertension.

Lability. Impairment of emotional control after brain damage; causes frequent, if brief, episodes of spontaneous laughing or crying with no obvious stimulus.

Lacunar stroke. Blockage of small vessels in the interior brain tissue caused by *hypertension* and/or *atherosclerosis*.

Lipid. *Fats, steroids,* phospholipids, and glycolipids; fat or fatlike substances.

Lipoprotein. Responsible for the transport of *lipids* in the blood, tissues, and fluids.

Malignant hypertension. Progressive *hypertension* that is usually due to *kidney* disease and is considered a medical emergency. Blood pressure readings consistent with malignant hypertension are higher than 200 millimeters of mercury.

Medulla oblongata. The part of the brain connected to the spine; responsible for the regulation of the heart, *blood vessels,* breathing, salivation, and swallowing.

Midbrain. Small portion of the brainstem.

Myocardial infarction. See *heart attack.*

Multiple risk phenomenon. The cumulative effect of various controllable habits and uncontrollable genetic traits on the development of disease.

Nephron. The unit of the *kidney* in which waste is removed from the body and urine is formed.

Nephrosclerosis. A hardening of the *arteries* and *arterioles* of the *kidney.*

Nervous system. The network of cells specialized to carry information by way of nerve impulses to and from various organ systems. The *central nervous system* is comprised of the brain and spinal cord; the peripheral nervous system is comprised of the remaining nerve *tissue* throughout the body.

Nicotine. A chemical substance derived from tobacco that affects blood pressure and pulse rate.

Norepinephrine. Also called noradrenaline. A hormone secreted by the adrenal gland. Raises blood pressure by constricting small *blood vessels* and increasing blood flow through the *coronary arteries.*

Obesity. The condition in which excess *fat* has accumulated in the body. Usually considered to be present when a person is 20 percent above the recommended weight for his or her height.

Pacer. The part of the heart that regulates the rate of its beat.

Pancreas. The *gland* situated behind the stomach that secretes a number of substances important for digestion, including the hormone *insulin.*

Parasympathetic nervous system. One of the two divisions of the *autonomic nervous system.* Frequently opposes the action of the *sympathetic nervous system*.

Paresis. Weakness of a muscle or group of muscles due to injury to the neuromuscular system.

Percutaneous transluminal angioplasty. Treatment for *atherosclerosis* and other arterial diseases involving threading a catheter with an inflatable balloon into the artery to remove blockage by flattening and widening the arterial opening.

Perception. The ability to receive, interpret, and use information through the sensory systems (vision, touch, taste, smell, and sound).

Platelet. Cellular component of the blood specifically involved in blood clotting. Platelets are much smaller than red or white blood cells.

Pons. The part of the brain that links the *medulla oblongata* and the *thalamus*.

Positron emission tomography (PET). A brain scan procedure in which the emission of radioactive particles injected into brain cells is measured by X ray.

Preeclampsia. A complication of pregnancy characterized by fluid retention and possibly kidney malfunction.

Progesterone. The female sex hormone secreted inside the ovary and other tissues. It causes the thickening of the uterine wall and other changes to prepare the body for conception.

Prothrombin. A substance in the blood that forms thrombin, an enzyme essential to blood coagulation.

Receptor. A cell or group of cells that detects changes in the body and triggers reactions in the nervous system.

Rehabilitation. The restoration of an individual after a disabling disease, injury, or other condition to the maximum of his or her physical, mental, social, spiritual, and vocational potentials.

Renal arteries. The two large arteries that supply blood to the kidney.

Renin. An enzyme found in the kidney that is transformed by other body tissues into *angiotensin*, which raises blood pressure in response to *stress*.

Retina. The layered lining of the eye that is light sensitive; the retina conveys images to the brain.

Risk factor. Those conditions associated with the increased likelihood of developing a disease. They include hereditary and environmental factors.

Sclerosis. An abnormal thickening or hardening of the *arteries* and other vessels.

Secondary hypertension. High blood pressure caused by a specific organ defect or disease.

Smooth muscle. Under the control of the *autonomic nervous system*, muscles that produce long-term, slow contractions such as occur in *blood vessels*.

Sodium. A mineral found in salt and essential body constituents. Controls the volume of fluids outside the cells. The amount of sodium in the body is controlled by the *kidneys*.

Spasm. Involuntary contraction of a muscle.

Sphygmomanometer. An instrument used to measure blood pressure.

Stenosis. A narrowing of an opening such as a *blood vessel*.

Steroid. Natural hormones or synthetic drugs that have many different effects.

Stress. Any factor that has an adverse effect on the body, physical or emotional.

Stroke. An interruption of the blood flow to the brain causing damage and loss of function. The primary disease is in the heart or blood vessels and the effect on the brain is secondary. Also referred to as a cerebrovascular accident (CVA).

Subarachnoid hemorrhage. A bleeding between the brain surface and one of the covering membranes. Typically caused by a ruptured *aneurysm*.

Sympathetic nervous system. The division of the *autonomic nervous system* responsible for such reflex actions as blood pressure, salivation, and digestion. Works in balance with the *parasympathetic nervous system*.

Systole. The contraction of the heart muscle. Systolic pressure is the greater of the two blood pressure readings.

Tachycardia. Abnormally rapid heartbeat.

Thalamus. One of two parts of the forebrain responsible for relaying all sensory messages that enter the brain.

Thromboembolism. The condition in which a part of a *thrombus*, formed at one point in the circulation, becomes unattached and lodges at another point, thereby blocking the vessel.

Thrombosis. The formation of a blood clot, called a *thrombus*, that partially or completely blocks *blood vessels*. The thrombosis may occur as the result of low flow in a narrowed vessel or it may result from embolus.

Thrombus. A blood clot.

Tissue. A group of cells or fibers that are specialized to perform a particular bodily function.

Transient ischemic attack (TIA). An interruption of blood supply to a part of the brain that causes temporary impairment of vision, speech, or movement. The interruption is usually brief, lasting a few minutes. If the interruption lasts for more than twenty-four hours it is called a stroke.

Triglyceride. The most common lipid found in fatty tissue; the form in which fat is stored in the body.

Vascular. Pertaining to or supplied with blood vessels.

Vasoconstrictor. An agent that causes the *blood vessels* to narrow, thereby causing a decrease in blood flow.

Vasodilator. An agent that causes the blood vessels to widen, thereby increasing blood flow.

Vasomotor nerve. Any nerve that controls the circulation of the blood through vessels by its action in the muscle fibers of the vessels or of the heart.

Veins. The vessels that carry deoxygenated blood from all parts of the body back to the heart.

Vertebral arteries. Major arteries leading to the brain.

Warfarin. An anticoagulant used to reduce the risk of blood clot formation and embolism.

Index

We Deliver!
And So Do These Bestsellers.

Bantam's Best in Health and Nutrition